The Care We Dream Of

The Care We Dream Of

Liberatory & Transformative Approaches to LGBTQ+ Health

ZENA SHARMAN

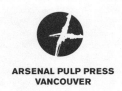

ARSENAL PULP PRESS
VANCOUVER

ARSENAL PULP PRESS
Suite 202 – 211 East Georgia St.
Vancouver, BC V6A 1Z6
Canada
arsenalpulp.com

The publisher gratefully acknowledges the support of the Canada Council for the Arts and the British Columbia Arts Council for its publishing program, and the Government of Canada, and the Government of British Columbia (through the Book Publishing Tax Credit Program), for its publishing activities.

 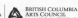 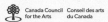

Arsenal Pulp Press acknowledges the xʷməθkʷəỳəm (Musqueam), Sḵwx̱wú7mesh (Squamish), and səlilwətaʔɬ (Tsleil-Waututh) Nations, custodians of the traditional, ancestral, and unceded territories where our office is located. We pay respect to their histories, traditions, and continuous living cultures and commit to accountability, respectful relations, and friendship.

Cover image description: The cover art of *The Care We Dream Of* is a painting by Tiaré Lani Kela Jung. The painting depicts a large bright moon with textures of pale yellows, pinks, blues, and purples mixed in with white. The background is a faded dark sky that lightens into orange by the bottom of the cover. Various plants local to the Pacific Northwest, including berries, flowers, and greenery, frame the moon. Purple berries drape down from the top of the cover, slightly overlapping the book's title, which is placed inside the moon in a calm, thin sans serif font. The subtitle is below the moon, in orange, against the dark night sky. The author's name, Zena Sharman, appears in a light cream over some of the foliage along the bottom of the cover. Below her name is dark grey text that reads, "Editor of the Lambda Literary Award–winning anthology *The Remedy*."

Cover and text design by Jazmin Welch
Cover and interior illustrations by Tiaré Lani Kela Jung
Edited by Shirarose Wilensky
Copy edited by Erin Parker
Proofread by Alison Strobel

Printed and bound in Canada

Library and Archives Canada Cataloguing in Publication:
Title: The care we dream of : liberatory & transformative approaches to LGBTQ+ health /
  Zena Sharman.
Names: Sharman, Zena, 1979– editor.
Description: Includes bibliographical references.
Identifiers: Canadiana (print) 2021022746X | Canadiana (ebook) 20210232374 |
  ISBN 9781551528601 (softcover) | ISBN 9781551528618 (HTML)
Subjects: LCSH: Sexual minorities—Medical care. | LCSH: Sexual minorities—
  Health and hygiene. | LCSH: Sexual minorities—Medical care—Literary collections. |
  LCSH: Sexual minorities—Health and hygiene—Literary collections. | LCSH: Sexual
  minorities' writings, Canadian. | CSH: Canadian literature (English)—21st century.
Classification: LCC RA564.9.S49 C37 2021 | DDC 362.1086/6—dc23

"the space is woven. multicolored bright patterns lovingly threaded together. when you touch them, you know that each piece was worn by someone who believed in this quilted moment, this soft vibrant welcoming space.

and you can feel that the hands that stitched this together stitched it with love and desire, creativity and connection. they laughed sometimes when they were stitching and cried sometimes as the memories came through. they were grateful to transform each memory into love. you can feel their presence as you put the fabric in your hands. as you begin weaving now."

—ALEXIS PAULINE GUMBS, *M ARCHIVE: AFTER THE END OF THE WORLD*

"A minimal definition of community might be this: folks who are reweaving."

—HIL MALATINO, *TRANS CARE*

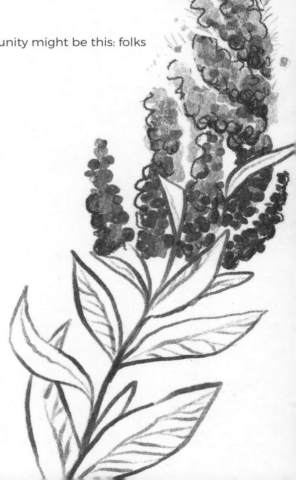

CONTENTS

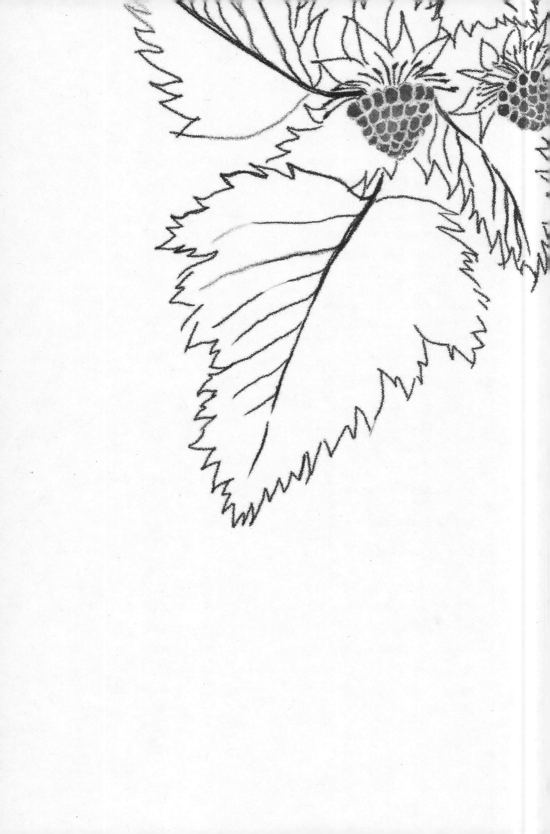

Introduction

Zena Sharman

This book began from a question: What if queer and trans people loved going to the doctor?

Questions can be a portal into possibilities we hadn't yet imagined. This deceptively simple question—*what if queer and trans people loved going to the doctor?*—was a kind of portal for me, because of how it gestured toward an audaciously different set of conditions from the ones we're in now.

When I ask other queer and trans people this question they usually laugh, roll their eyes, or make a face that tells me just how unfathomable the idea of loving going to the doctor is to them. But then something changes. As they contemplate what it would mean to feel this way, their facial expressions shift. Their eyes light up and their bodies relax a little. I know because mine does, too. There's something potent about this moment of shared imagining, even if we aren't picturing the same thing.

Think about it: What if *you* loved going to the doctor?

I'm curious: What's the first thing that comes to mind when you contemplate this question? How does it feel in your body? Maybe you're already rolling your eyes at me or you instinctively put up a shield to protect yourself from potential harm. Sit with this question for a moment longer if you can. What kinds of possibilities begin to unfold for you as you let yourself imagine what it would take to be able to answer yes?

When I asked myself this question, it led me to other questions: What if queer and trans people had the resources we needed to create and sustain our own community-led forms of care and healing in ways that are expansively available to everyone who wants them? What if we could always trust in getting health care that felt good, accessible, and even pleasurable, wherever and whenever we needed it? What if it felt safe enough to bring our whole selves into the process? What if health care felt healing and helped us flourish?

What if all health care providers and healers genuinely honoured and valued queer and trans people, worked collaboratively with us, and trusted in our expert knowledge of our own bodies? What if health and healing were widely understood not as individual responsibilities but as processes that happen collectively in communities? What if all health care and healing was built on a foundation of anti-racism and disability justice? What if the care we received was rooted in a commitment to our liberation and the liberation of all people?

What if?

This book is about finding our way toward being able to answer yes to these questions while reckoning with how and why the health system isn't serving us and our communities. It's an invitation to practise dreaming beyond this system by imagining more liberatory and transformative approaches to LGBTQ+ health.

When I say "health," I don't mean in the limiting, ableist, and judgment-laden way this word often gets used. This isn't a book that asks you to "make healthy choices" or conform to a normative ideal of health. Rather, I'm interested in reaching back to the roots of the word "health," which invoke wholeness, healing, happiness, safety, and sacredness.

Sociologist Bobbie Harro defines liberation as "the practice of love," a love "big enough to encompass all society, and active enough to transform it."[1] To me, liberatory health care means conspiring to change a fundamentally harmful system in ways that centre the leadership, needs, and priorities of the people in our communities who bear the brunt of systemic oppression.[2] It sometimes means divesting from the health system altogether and creating something different. This isn't about quick fixes or easily measurable outcomes; it's an everyday commitment sustained over time. As Dean Spade reminds us, this kind of work is "about practice and process rather than arrival at a singular point of 'liberation.'"[3]

To transform is to change. It is to bring creativity, imagination, and the full force of our dreams to these changes. It is a reminder we can dream differently and expect more. At its heart, *The Care We Dream Of* is a spell of transformation. This book is a calling out, a calling in, and a call to action. It is a refusal, an antidote, and a holding to account. It is a perversion, and a space of infinite possibilities. It's an offering to my queer and trans ancestors and the descendants who'll come after us. *The Care We Dream Of* is both a loving invitation and an urgent demand to leave no one behind as we dream a more liberated future into being.

DREAMING TOGETHER AND DEMANDING MORE

The Care We Dream Of is not quite an essay collection, not quite an anthology. In this way, it joins a lineage of books that defy easy categorization, along with titles like Harsha Walia's *Undoing Border Imperialism* or adrienne maree brown's *Pleasure Activism*. I feel a kinship with these books because of the ways they demonstrate collectivity and multiplicity, and in how they emerge from communities and webs of relationships.

The Care We Dream Of reflects my commitment to collectivity, and my belief that there are as many visions for liberatory and transformative health and healing as there are queer and trans people.

That's why this book weaves together my essays on topics like queering health and healing, transforming the health system, kinship, aging, and death with stories, poetry, and nonfiction by Alexander McClelland and Zoë Dodd, Blyth Barnow, Carly Boyce, jaye simpson, Jillian Christmas, Joshua Wales, Kai Cheng Thom, Leah Lakshmi Piepzna-Samarasinha, and Sand C. Chang. It also includes interviews with Anita "Durt" O'Shea (of St. James Infirmary), Dawn Serra, Hannah Kia, Ronica Mukerjee, and Sean Saifa Wall. It's a joy and a privilege to be able to share their words with you.

The writing and interviews in this book explore a range of topics and themes. One of these through lines is the practice of reclaiming and redefining healing, as you'll find in pieces like Leah Lakshmi Piepzna-Samarasinha's "Cripping Healing" or jaye simpson's "the seven sacred ways of healing." Blyth Barnow shows us how queer do-it-yourself ritual can be a means of holding ourselves and each other even in the face of our deepest grief and heartbreaking losses like a beloved friend dying by suicide. In "seed," Jillian Christmas offers us a plant-inspired meditation on growing that carries us forward and backward in time. She reminds us, "You are your own medicine, Beloved, you already hold the seed to whatever healing you seek."

Another theme running through *The Care We Dream Of* is the politicization of health and healing. Nurse practitioner Ronica Mukerjee explores what this can look like in the context of a health care worker's own practice, challenging health care workers to put themselves on the line in service of liberation. Anita "Durt" O'Shea shows us what this can look like at the level of a whole clinic through the example of St. James Infirmary, the first occupational health and safety clinic in the United States run by sex workers for sex workers. Drawing on an analysis of care work, Kai Cheng Thom invites therapists to question their positionality and assumptions about sex work. She calls for solidarity among care workers while also holding the so-called "helping professions" to account for the harm and violence they often perpetuate against sex workers.

Dawn Serra's interview invites us to imagine the liberatory possibilities inherent in pleasure-centred health care while reckoning with the barriers that stand in the way of realizing them. It's a reminder of the importance of pleasure in a world where we're often conditioned to withstand pain. In an essay exploring body liberation and weight inclusivity in health care, Sand C. Chang challenges us to redefine disordered eating to be inclusive of queer and trans people and depicts a future where there is enough space for *every* body to thrive. These pathways are important for envisioning and creating the care we dream of; we can find inspiration and guidance in history and in what people are doing today. In "Borrowed Wisdom," Carly Boyce shares lessons for suicide intervention rooted in their learnings from community, history, and their own lived and embodied experiences.

Intersex activist Sean Saifa Wall offers strategies and tactics for change grounded in learnings from Black- and people of colour–led movements for intersex justice. His work, like mine and that of many contributors to this book, is rooted in a deep commitment to ancestors and descendants. As he puts it, "I'm planting seeds for future generations of activists. Whatever they want to do with the harvest is up to them." Alexander McClelland and Zoë Dodd offer us approaches to responding to Hepatitis C and HIV grounded in anarchism. They highlight "mutual aid, spontaneity, trust, and collaboration" as key tenets of this work, tracing historical lineages of activism as they envision forms future responses might take.

It can sometimes feel challenging for queer and trans people to imagine futures for ourselves; aging might feel impossible, and death might feel scary, inevitable, or both. Hannah Kia invites us to consider the emancipatory potential of aging while reckoning with the complexities of getting older in a context of neoliberalism. Drawing on his experiences as a palliative care physician, Joshua Wales uses fiction to depict death as an intimate act of solidarity between doctor and patient, one that intentionally queers the institutional space of the hospital. I hope these pieces, alongside my own writing on aging and death, might offer you generative, encouraging, and perhaps unexpected possibilities as you contemplate their relevance to your life. Creating this book has shifted my own perspective on aging and death and vastly expanded my sense of what queer and trans health and healing can look like at every stage of our lives.

The Care We Dream Of is a book deeply rooted in community and collaboration, in that I'm connected to every person who is part of this book through an interconnected web of queer relationships that spans continents. This book centres community knowledge, expertise, and action because the most important and sophisticated things I know about LGBTQ+ health I learned from, in, and with my community and through my queer body, not from a doctor or a textbook.

It reflects what I've learned and how my own thinking about queer and trans health has shifted in the years since my last book, *The Remedy: Queer and Trans Voices on Health and Health Care*, was published in 2016. *The Remedy* was a collection of stories by queer and trans people about their experiences as patients, health care providers, and providers-in-training. They vividly portrayed the harmful impacts of non-affirming health care and offered joyful glimpses of what affirming, accessible, LGBTQ+-centred care can look like. The stories in *The Remedy* validated queer and trans people's experiences, offered health care providers new insights on how to care for us, and were a collective call to action for systems change. Five years later, readers of *The Remedy* keep telling me they read it and then passed it on to someone else or bought a second copy and immediately gave it away. I cherish this image of the book, travelling from person to person, doing its work of change.

What *The Remedy* didn't do was offer readers an answer to the question, "Now what?" *The Care We Dream Of* is my attempt to answer this question by merging the practical with liberatory imaginings about what queer and trans health care could be, grounded in historical examples, present-day experiments, and dreams of the future. It isn't a comprehensive guide to every LGBTQ+ health issue or topic—there are gaps, and this book could easily have been twice as long.

I started working on *The Care We Dream Of* in the summer of 2019. Although it predates the COVID-19 pandemic, this book was fundamentally shaped by the experience of creating it during a time when the harms and violence of racism, ableism, ageism, fatphobia, and other forms of systemic oppression were so evident. Living and writing in this context has filled me with grief and rage and challenged me to be bolder in the demands I make of the health system, and of myself. It has pushed me to embody a more radical spirit, take bigger risks in service of collective liberation, and to learn to dream differently in service of a more expansive, imaginative vision of queer and trans health and healing.

NAVIGATING THE GAP BETWEEN OUR DREAMS AND OUR REALITIES

The truth is, there's a big gap between the care I dream of and where we are now. Hardly any queer or trans person I know loves going to the doctor, and it's not only because of the long waits for appointments, scratchy paper gowns, or outdated magazines in the waiting room. It's because of an accumulation of experiences that leave us convinced we won't be treated with dignity, kindness, and understanding when we access health care. For many LGBTQ+ people, spaces like the clinic, the emergency department, or the therapist's office feel scary, traumatic, and violent instead of being havens of safety, care, trust, and healing.

As queer and trans people living at the intersections of many identities, we remember all the times we've been called by the wrong name or pronoun by a care provider, were met with suspicion or disbelief when we tried explaining where we are hurting and why, or given inadequate pain relief because someone wrongly believes Indigenous, Black, or Brown bodies deserve less pain relief or feel less pain than white bodies do. We remember feeling like we can't talk openly about drug use, sex work, or suicidal ideation because we're afraid we'll be judged, stigmatized, and at risk of being surveilled, criminalized, or incarcerated in a psych ward or a jail. We feel like we can't show our whole selves to the people whose job it is to care for us.

Many LGBTQ+ people associate accessing health care with feeling invisible or too visible or like nobody understands us, our bodies, our relationships, and who we call family. Far too many of us can't get the care we need because we don't have enough money or we lack health insurance, we're incarcerated or undocumented, how and where that care is offered is inaccessible to people with disabilities, or we live in communities where it's difficult or impossible to access the care we need locally.

All this rolls up into a picture of inadequate, inaccessible, and sometimes harmful health care. Data from Canada, the United States, and Europe tells a similar story: LGBTQ+ people experience discrimination and barriers to health care, including outright denial of care. Trans people consistently report the highest rates of health care discrimination—around 20 to 30 percent of trans people compared to around 10 percent of lesbian, gay, bisexual, or queer people.[4] Research has shown that bisexual people, who experience biphobia, stigma, and erasure both within and outside the LGBTQ+ community, are less likely to tell health care providers about their bisexuality.[5] Black, Indigenous, and people of colour; disabled people; poor people; and fat people also report higher rates of health care discrimination and mistreatment by care providers. LGBTQ+ people studying to become health care providers or who work as health care providers face stigma and discrimination at school and work, experiences exacerbated by the racism, ableism, and sexual violence so pervasive in these spaces.[6]

Queer and trans people instinctively brace ourselves for the impacts of discrimination—I notice it in how I steel myself before seeing a new health care provider. My shoulders tense up and my body stiffens as I physically and emotionally armour up to mitigate against the possibility of harm. Many LGBTQ+ people know what it's like to deliberately avoid or postpone medical care, preventative screening, and trips to the clinic or the emergency department because of fear of discrimination. Trans, nonbinary, and gender-diverse people face additional barriers to care, sometimes forgoing needed health care as a strategy to protect themselves against the harms of the transphobia, transmisogyny, and cisnormativity so prevalent in many health care settings.[7]

When we do access health care, we strategize about which parts of ourselves to conceal or reveal to be considered credible and worthy of care. In an essay called "On Being Bipolar," writer andrea bennett tells the story of being a pregnant nonbinary person with a history of mental illness. During their pregnancy, they chose not to come out as nonbinary to their OB/GYN and other health care providers. Explaining their decision, bennett writes,

> I had a very strong urge to be as candid as possible about being bipolar so that I could be streamed into emergency mental health care if it became necessary. While being candid, though, I also wanted to appear as stable, as *normal*, as possible ... I did not know if I could afford to be non-binary and bipolar. So I compromised.[8]

I am dreaming of a world where these kinds of compromises are unnecessary.

I am dreaming of a world where LGBTQ+ people can be uncompromising in our expectation that we can always access health care and healing with dignity, safety, and the joy that comes with being honoured and valued in the fullness of our identities and ways of relating. I am dreaming of a world where LGBTQ+ people love going to the doctor, nurse, counsellor, midwife, massage therapist, traditional healer, or any other practitioner we see, and where health care providers work under conditions that enable them to flourish while caring for their patients and clients. I am dreaming of a world where LGBTQ+ people who are Indigenous, Black, Latinx, Asian, and/or from other communities of colour can access healing and health care that centres and honours their intersecting identities and cultures.

I am dreaming of a world where LGBTQ+ communities are lavishly resourced to organize community-led, peer-based healing, care, and mutual aid for each other. I am dreaming of a world with an abundance of LGBTQ+ elders, where we are surrounded by queer and trans people who are old and thriving, living alongside children being raised by families and communities who love them for the perfection of exactly who they are, honour their bodily sovereignty, and joyfully affirm however they choose to express their genders or sexualities, at every stage of their lives.

This is the care I dream of. This is the world I am working to help create.

I want to know: What is the care *you* dream of, and how can we work together to bring it into being?

SURVIVE, DREAM, BUILD

The Care We Dream Of is grounded in a lineage of queer and trans health activism that spans generations. Our communities have a history of fighting, organizing, loving, and dreaming the care we need into being, often informally and with few resources, and of holding unjust systems accountable for all the ways they've failed us. This dual reality—navigating the system that exists to survive long enough to build something new—feels inherently queer to me. We're a community accustomed to doing what we need to do to survive, to holding unjust systems accountable, and changing them from outside and from within, while simultaneously imagining and creating the systems and structures we need not just to survive, but to flourish.

Myrl Beam captures this idea in his book *Gay, Inc.*, in a case study of the Trans Youth Support Network, a Minneapolis, Minnesota–based group he was part of. Taking inspiration from Dean Spade, Beam writes, "We decided [our] work was to support trans folks in *surviving* the systems with which they must engage, create the space necessary to *dream* of another world, and then gather the resources and power necessary to *build* it."[9] Many LGBTQ+ people are doing the work of surviving, dreaming, and building every day, both within and outside the health system.

This is evident in histories of mutual aid within the LGBTQ+ community, like the community-led gay health clinics established as an alternative to the mainstream health system in the 1970s and subsequent community health organizing and activism during the AIDS crisis. It's evident in spaces like Street Transvestite Action Revolutionaries (STAR House), the first LGBTQ+ youth shelter in North America founded in 1970 by Marsha P. Johnson and Sylvia Rivera, activists and organizers who were trans women of colour and sex workers. Johnson and Rivera's STAR manifesto, also written in 1970, centred on nine demands. They included "The end to all exploitive practices of doctors and psychiatrists who work in the field of transvestites" and "Transvestites and gay street people and all oppressed people should have free education, health care, clothing, food, transportation, and housing."[10]

These histories are intertwined with those of other communities who created their own radical alternatives to the mainstream health system, like the Black Panthers and the Young Lords, as well as within the women's health movement, the reproductive justice movement, the disability justice movement, and among groups like psychiatric survivors, sex workers, and people who use drugs. (I explore some of these examples in more detail alongside others in the chapter called "Regrowth in Ruins.")

In the face of systemic challenges that can feel daunting and overwhelming, I find it comforting to know that we have ancestors and lineages to learn from. I take inspiration from these lineages and also feel accountable to them as I look backward and forward in time. What tools, strategies, ideas, and possibilities will we leave behind for the queer and trans people who come after us? What medicines will we offer them? How will we be remembered by our descendants?

LINEAGES, LIVED EXPERIENCES, AND THE LIMITS OF MY KNOWLEDGE

While I was working on *The Care We Dream Of*, my cousin sent me a photo of my mom, Lynne, and me taken in the summer of 1987 when I was eight years old. It's a black and white picture of a group of women and children silently parading down a city sidewalk. The women are wearing strange and elaborate dresses adorned with tea bags, dried moss, dead insects, condoms, and intrauterine devices, their images reflected back to them by a plate glass store window. My mother is in the middle of the group wearing a white dress and a gas mask; my small face is visible behind her right shoulder. I remember feeling both thrilled and mortified to be part of something so publicly weird. A rounded silver-and-white city bus passes by our group. I can't see inside it, but I'm sure the passengers were gawking at the strange sight on Red River Road.

In the foreground of the photo is Rebecca Belmore, a member of the Lac Seul First Nation (Anishinaabe), who led the procession. Now a renowned multidisciplinary artist, she describes this 1987 performance as one of her foundational early works. Belmore wears a sculptural gown called *Rising to the Occasion*, which she designed to draw attention to the impacts of colonization on Indigenous women. Modelled after a Victorian tea gown, the front of the full skirt is burgundy and grey-blue velvet and cream brocade. The back is a bustle made to look like a beaver dam, a tangle of branches and sticks "with royalty memorabilia and trade objects (silver flatware, kitsch souvenir mugs, and so on)" caught in its dense weave.[11] The bodice is beaded with flowers and adorned by a breastplate made of bone china saucers, topped off with buckskin epaulets. Belmore wears a headpiece with two tall black braided ropes standing on end, their edges frayed. An eagle feather is tied to one braid, a piece of broken saucer to the other. An antler curves around Belmore's forehead, and if you look closely, you'll notice a small picture of Queen Elizabeth wrapped around her headband.

The procession, called *Twelve Angry Crinolines*, took place in Thunder Bay, the small city in Northwestern Ontario where I grew up. The city is on the traditional lands of the Fort William First Nation, signatory to the Robinson-Superior Treaty of 1850, on the traditional territory of the Anishinaabeg and the Métis. In the 1800s, Thunder Bay was a hub of the colonial fur trade; it later became home to a tourist attraction then called Old Fort William, a reconstruction of the original fur trading post.

In 1987, royal newlyweds Prince Andrew and Sarah Ferguson, the Duke and Duchess of York, visited Thunder Bay as part of an official tour. While there, they visited the fort and paddled a birchbark canoe for an audience of thrilled locals. When asked about *Rising to the Occasion*, Belmore remarked, "The royals came to our city for a handful of hours as performers replaying colonial history complete with birchbark canoes and a fake fort. This was incredibly absurd to me. What to wear for such an absurd occasion?"[12]

My mother conceived of *Twelve Angry Crinolines* as a protest against the royal visit. Earlier that year, it was revealed that five developmentally disabled members of the royal family, cousins to the queen, had been secretly incarcerated in an asylum for forty years and declared dead.[13] In an interview about the performance protest, my mother said, "We would like to know why these five women were locked away." She continued, "We look at the royal family as a corporation. We're drawing parallels between the incarceration of these women and the peripheral status of female artists in Canada, particularly in an isolated community like Thunder Bay."[14] She invited women artists involved with Definitely Superior, the local artist-run centre she helped found, to cocreate the procession, which was followed by a video performance and a "mad tea party" at the gallery.

My mom was an artist, activist, and survivor who was disabled by the abuse, violence, and torture she suffered as a child. Her beloved younger sister, my aunt Wendy, is developmentally disabled and was institutionalized in the 1950s, though she later transitioned to community living as part of the deinstitutionalization movement. Wendy's experiences are part of what prompted my mother to protest the royal family's actions, though her solidarity with incarcerated people went beyond her sibling. My mother's own experiences of violence made her intensely mistrustful of the state and anyone who sought to subjugate another person's body/mind. They also made her passionate about connecting with, fighting for, and supporting other survivors.

My mom wore her hair in two long silver braids, had a wardrobe of plaid shirts from the thrift store and a wry sense of humour, and exuded a quiet strength. She smoked menthol cigarettes and drank coffee all day long in her kitchen-turned-home-office-turned-activist-command-central. She knew exactly how much everything cost because we were on welfare and money was always tight. My mom raised me on her own and loved me fiercely. She taught me to respect and listen deeply to children, believe them, and delight in their creativity, qualities I instinctively bring to my own parenting because of her. My mom died in 2014 and is an ancestor I've held close through the process of working on this book. When I think about who I am, where I come from, and why I do what I do, I always begin with my mother, Lynne.

My mom taught me from an early age what it looks like to organize in opposition to unjust systems and how important it is to document and share people's stories, experiences, and survival strategies. Much of her work centred on women and children who were survivors of abuse, violence, and torture, including at the hands of violent systems like residential schools, foster care, prisons, and psychiatric institutions. She lived in Thunder Bay for nearly thirty years and cultivated deep and sustained relationships with Indigenous people there, which foundationally shaped her world view and activism.

In the 1990s and 2000s, my mother formed advocacy groups for survivors, creating a zine-like journal of their stories and drawings that she circulated across North America. She organized conferences that connected survivors with each other and taught therapists to do a better job of caring for them. She supported and advocated for people who were facing sentencing, were currently incarcerated, or had recently been released from jail or prison. She cofounded a memorial walk for missing and murdered Indigenous women, girls, and Two-Spirit people, and kept a meticulous archive of stories documenting what happened to them at a time when the government steadfastly refused to acknowledge the scope of this colonial violence. (This archive of stories is now housed at the University of Manitoba.) My mom was an activist who did the majority of this work without pay, from her kitchen table, with and for her community.

Working on this book pushed me to look closer at my mom's legacy of activism and how growing up as her daughter influenced me. The more I learn about everything she did, the more I wish she were still alive so I could ask her about it. What I know for certain is that I am who I am because I am Lynne Moss Sharman's daughter. I've had a photo of her smiling down at me throughout the process of working on this book. When I look at it, I'm reminded of who I come from and what it taught me about art, activism, and holding unjust systems accountable, working alongside my community, and fighting like hell for a better world.

Writing about health and health care is as much an embodied and relational experience as it is an intellectual exercise. It feels important to situate myself in terms of who I am, where I come from, and who I'm in relationship with. I'm a white queer femme in my early forties who's coparenting a toddler with three other queer people including my partner, who's nonbinary. I've been a caregiver to my loved ones, both for my queer chosen family and for my mother at the end of her life. I think about aging and death a lot more than I did when I was younger and am compelled by questions about interdependence and fostering intergenerational queer and trans communities. You'll notice these themes woven throughout *The Care We Dream Of*.

I'm a queer and trans health advocate and activist, writer, and PhD-trained health researcher. LGBTQ+ health advocacy and writing are my passion, my purpose, and a way I can be of service to my community, but they've never been my full-time job. I pay my bills with day jobs in the health research sector and write on the side. This book was written in the early mornings before work, on weekends, and during my vacations, while the three adults I'm coparenting with picked up the domestic slack for me. I wrote while my kid napped and at 5:30 a.m. with a cup of coffee at my side. I say this because of how it evokes my mom's legacy for me, and because it feels important to signal what the process of creating this book looked like.

I wrote this book in Vancouver, British Columbia, a city I've lived in for the past twenty years. Two decades feels long to me, but it's a tiny fraction of time compared to the thousands of years Vancouver has been the traditional, ancestral, and unceded shared territory of the xʷməθkʷəy̓əm (Musqueam), Sḵwx̱wú7mesh (Squamish), and səlilwəta?ɬ (Tsleil-Waututh) Nations. As a white queer person whose ancestors came from Scotland and Ireland to live in Canada as settlers on stolen Indigenous lands, I'm in an ongoing process of learning and practising what it means to be a respectful visitor and guest on lands that don't belong to me and that have been stewarded by Indigenous peoples since time immemorial.[15]

I am working to understand what it means to be in an accountable, reciprocal, loving relationship with the land instead of treating it as a lifeless commodity to be extracted from and used. I'm thinking about a conversation I had recently with a friend of mine who is Indigenous, and who told me rematriating land to the stewardship and care of the Indigenous peoples it was stolen from is fundamental to any policy solution she would offer in response to the health and other disparities Indigenous people face today as a result of colonization. As Eve Tuck and K. Wayne Yang remind us, "Decolonization is not a metaphor."[16]

My knowledge of LGBTQ+ health is both rooted in and limited by who I am. I come to this work through my body, and with the knowledge that my body doesn't bear the brunt of the health disparities that disproportionately affect the LGBTQ+ community. I'm cis, thin, and nondisabled. Although I grew up in poverty, as an adult I'm middle class and economically secure and I have stable housing, two things that were lacking in my childhood and adolescence. I live in a big city where I have access to a diverse range of health care providers, some of whom have training in LGBTQ+ health, in a country with universal health care. In short, although I'm a queer woman, I move through the world with a lot of privilege and ease. This limits what I know—and what I can know or understand—about queer and trans health, and it complicates my positioning as an expert.

It's one of the reasons I invited other people to contribute their writing and ideas to this book. I tried to create *The Care We Dream Of* in a way that acknowledges and is accountable to the limits of my knowledge and expertise, and I know I made mistakes. I will endeavour to learn from them and be accountable for them. This feels especially important for me as someone whose evolving understanding of LGBTQ+ health has been strongly influenced by disability justice, healing justice, reproductive justice, fat liberation, transformative justice, and prison industrial complex abolitionism. These are lineages of thought, activism, cultural and community work led by and rooted in communities of Black, Indigenous, and people of colour, many of whom are queer, trans, and/or disabled.

I'm committed to respecting and acknowledging these lineages in ways that don't replicate the patterns of theft and appropriation that are integral to white supremacy. It's one of the reasons why I make a deliberate practice of citing my sources—this isn't just an academic convention; it's a politicized act of recognition that these ideas aren't mine. What seems new or innovative to me may be reflective of ways of knowing and being that span generations, and I am not entitled to claim every idea as my own. I acknowledge that despite my best intentions, I have probably engaged in acts of appropriation as I wrote this book. It's a reflection of the subtle, insidious conditioning into whiteness I've been taught all my life and am in an ongoing process of unlearning. As a gesture of reciprocity and reparations, I will donate at least half of all of my earnings from this book to groups and organizations focused on the healing and liberation of queer and trans people who are Black, Indigenous, and people of colour.

INVITATIONS: WAYS TO READ THIS BOOK

As you read *The Care We Dream Of*, I invite you to reflect on your own knowledge and assumptions about LGBTQ+ health and health care and how those might shape your perspective and the kinds of possibilities you're able to imagine. Consider reading from a place of curiosity. You don't have to agree with everything in these pages, but I hope you'll be open to the possibility of being changed by the experience of engaging with this book. For those of you who have roles where you also are positioned as experts in other people's health—maybe you're a health care provider or a researcher—I encourage you to read from a place of humility and a willingness to have your authority challenged by the ideas and perspectives in this book.

Reading a book like this one isn't a neutral experience. For some of you, it might confront or challenge your understanding of LGBTQ+ health and health care. I created this book as a deliberate attempt to shift people's perceptions and as a way to gather knowledge that is rarely taught in formal education about health and health care. I wrote it as a balm for queer and trans folks who carry deep wounds inflicted by our engagement with health care providers and the health system. It's a survival guide, yes, but it's also an act of radical imagination. I want us to dream a different future into being together.

Some parts of the book may resonate with you more than others. You get to decide how you engage with *The Care We Dream Of*: maybe you want to read it chronologically, from start to finish, or dive into specific pieces or sections that feel especially relevant or interesting to you right now. Maybe you'll devour it in one sitting or savour it slowly. You also get to decide when to skip over something or pause to take care of yourself when you read stuff that feels triggering. This book is ultimately about imagining radical possibilities for our health and healing, but it covers some difficult topics along the way, like racism, colonialism, homophobia, transphobia, transmisogyny, ableism, trauma, violence, suicide, and death. It's why, after contemplating the possibility and talking it through with a mentor, I opted to not include detailed content warnings for this book. The truth is, this whole book might feel triggering, which is a reflection of what we're up against and why systemic transformation is both necessary and possible.

You'll find questions throughout this book because I write from a place of curiosity, and because questions are a way into creativity and expanding our sense of possibilities. I invite you to take time to reflect on the questions that feel most compelling or powerful to you. This book is an act of radical imagination and I want us to dream together.

Early in the process of writing *The Care We Dream Of*, I created an intention I've returned to again and again while working on it: *Let this book, and the process of creating it, be a spell of healing and transformation, rooted in love.*

This book is an offering of love threaded through with rage, grief, and a fierce commitment to the queer and trans community. I hope it offers you some of the medicine you need and helps you be with your own grief, rage, and fear for yourself and the future. I hope it inspires you to dream different possibilities for queer and trans health into being, both for us and in service of a more liberated and joyful future for all our descendants.

seed

Jillian Christmas

On the phone today, my father tells me about his relationship with my maternal grandmother, *we were gardeners together*, he says. He still watches over the plant they took turns tending—it has kept him company for twenty years. One day he will slip a clipping in the mail for me, defying all physical distance and braiding my hands into the lineage of quiet gardeners who have kept it safe. My father's mother still pushes her 101-year wise and nimble fingers into the soil to pull up the fruits of her labours and the bulk of her meals. For my mother it has always been flowers. There is a honeybee in her chest and it points her like a compass toward sweetness. We are none of us farmers; we are lovely and complicated things, quietly growing, dipping our roots into the damp darkness, and throwing blossoms into the sky.

When the stress of my daily work wore my body into a thin suit I dragged from bed to boardroom, and the sharpness of the world began to show up in ways I had never expected—two round coins of smooth flesh pinned like new blooms to my temples and a body covered in rose-coloured hives—there was no choice but to surrender to slowing. I held my own body like a wilted plant, I fed myself regularly and spoke to me the way I'd witnessed my grandmother baby her beloved banana plant. *You are a good thing, a sweet thing. Look how precious you are.*

When we are wealthy with wisdom, we never stop growing, tending to what in us needs attention and deserves kindness.

A large part of my continuous healing journey has been a practice of working with flowers, a medicine that is sometimes found in slow teas, or lavish body adornment. A medicine that reminds me that I am at every moment a seed, a root, a growing thing, with the possibility to stretch deeper and further than I can imagine.

What follows here is an offering of meditation, a collection of lessons and questions and imaginings that have unfolded from my explorations in growing. My hope is that you will share this, read it aloud to a loved one, ask a friend to read it to you, record it in your own voice and see what blossoms between your lips. You are your own medicine, Beloved, you already hold the seed to whatever healing you seek.

BELOVED: A MEDITATION

soil/ seed/ water/ fruit

Inside of you   there is a wild garden growing
sweet fruit of the seed buried deep   and still
Blooming; strength of vines longer and stronger
than any trial or sacrifice   you are a wonder
You are the gift   do you remember the last time
you heard magic whispered   in your own name
Will you kneel at your own altar   lay flowers
at your own feet?   Beloved

Picture yourself as a small child, safe and loved. Only you know what age you are. You are wrapped in your favourite blanket; your hair is styled just the way you like it. Your favourite song is swimming through your head and there is a sweet smile on your face.

seed/ water/ fruit/ soil

You can feel the energy of youth buzzing inside of you. Your wiggly toes, your attention, wild. Around you there is a large open field filled with dandelions, they stretch out wide in every direction, bright yellow under a big blue and cotton-candy-pink sky. Can you smell the air? Can you hear the chirring of small birds and the little bugs they are chasing? You sit down, feel the crinkle of grass between your toes. Stretch long so that you are lying on your back, dandelions now reaching up from behind you like miniature fur-lined skyscrapers. It's warm outside and suddenly it starts to drizzle. Warm flecks of water dust your face. Your fingers twirl into the grass and reach to pull up a dandelion between your fingers. This one a puffball of white. A perfect globe. You take in the deepest breath. Deep deep down to your toes. Bring the flower to your lips and exhale a dazzling snow that feathers down around you, twinkling in the soft light. You can hear someone calling your name and it sounds like a bell between their lips.

THE CARE WE DREAM OF

water/ fruit/ soil/ seed

Beloved, picture yourself a teenager. You are standing at the lip of the ocean. Can you see your bare feet? Can you smell the air filling with salt and seaweed and the great deep? The waves pull out and away they rush back toward you, submerging your toes in warm water. Each time the water comes, your toes dig deeper, the sand crumbling under your wriggling feet. It is the middle of the day. There is sun on every corner of your face. Notice how the water brings new life each time it comes. Notice how you stretch into the warmth of it. How it expands both in and outside of you. Your whole body pulsing. Alive and growing more vibrant each moment. Hear the waves, constant. Suddenly there is a laughter that mixes in with the pulsing waves. It may take a moment before you realize it is coming out of you. Swim in the sound of your laughing. Bathe and sun and bathe and sun and soak it all in. You have arrived.

fruit/ soil/ seed/ water

Beloved, picture yourself at the peak of your growing. What does your smile look like here? What relief pours over you as you look at the fruits of all of your labours? The dreams you set out to accomplish are spread out before you. A feast of dreams, where kin come to gather, marvel, and celebrate in your abundance. There is a beautiful vessel in your hands, resplendent and overflowing. As you bring it to your lips, fresh jewels of pomegranate burst between your teeth, sweetness erupting on your tongue. Can you feel yourself filling with the promise of enough? Here young ones come to seek your counsel, and still, there are mentors, friends, and teachers who guide your way forward. A long path stretches out behind you and an equally long and surprising road unfolds ahead. Everything is possible. What do you want here? What do you seek in your ripeness? What desires have you forgotten? Outgrown? What new curiosities bristle under your skin?

soil/ seed/ water/ fruit

Beloved, picture yourself, quiet and still. Your eyes lightly closed; your metronome is set by the time of your own breath. Nowhere to go rushing. No to-do list to check. Just the rhythm of your body. Just the sound of gentle birds outside your window. Occasionally you hear the wave of a new voice, a loved one come to surround and hold you, then another. Occasionally a flood of energy runs through you and you are lit up; you save your best stories for these moments. If they are lucky and wise, they slow down a while to listen. And there you outstretch a spiral of stories. A long life of dreams and questions and wishes. You remember for them a small child alone and deeply loved, singing to themself a wisdom born in small bones. Paint them the picture, blue and pink skies, a feeling of so much freedom. Fingers in the long grass. A dandelion pressed to your lips. A long calm exhale.

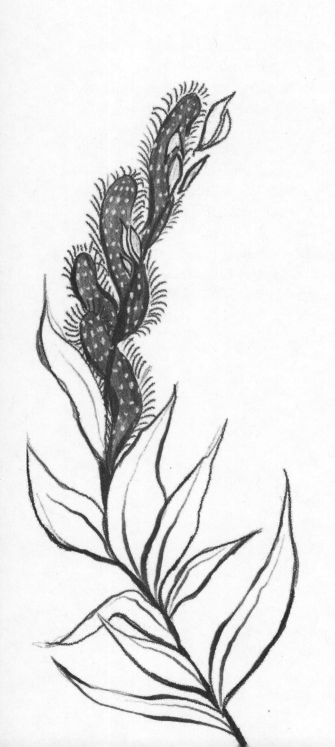

Queer Alchemy

Perverting the Health System, Fighting to Win

Zena Sharman

PERVERT IS A VERB: FUCKING TO WIN

In my bedroom there is a small gold hexagonal mirror painted with the words, "Every Time We Fuck, We Win." It was made by Lex Non Scripta, a nonbinary artist and organizer who created it as part of a series of typographic paintings centred on queer history and activism.[17] I bought it on Christmas Eve in 2013, as a gift to myself. At the time, I understood that the words were inspired by the manifesto of an activist group called Queer Nation, but I knew little about the history and context in which it was written. This mirror has had a prominent place in my bedroom for years, a declaration glinting warmly at anyone who pays close enough attention to the details to notice. But until recently, I hadn't given much thought to what it meant to see myself reflected in those words or where they came from.

The Queer Nation manifesto was written in 1990. The group was founded by Tom Blewitt, Alan Klein, Michelangelo Signorile, and Karl Soehnlein, AIDS activists from the New York chapter of the AIDS Coalition To Unleash Power (ACT UP), in response to an escalation of violence toward and persistent discrimination against LGBTQ+ people.[18] In 1990, Queer Nation marched with the ACT UP contingent in the New York City pride parade, handing out copies of their manifesto printed on pieces of newsprint titled "Queers Read This!" and "I Hate Straights!"

Earlier that year, a hundred ACT UP members were arrested for protesting the US Centers for Disease Control's narrow definition of AIDS, which excluded women and people who used injection drugs.[19] Several months later, a thousand people stormed the headquarters of the National Institutes of Health (NIH). They staged a die-in, planting cardboard tombstones across the NIH lawn and demanding more AIDS treatments and expansion of clinical trials to include women and people of colour.[20]

They scattered the ashes of their dead on the White House lawn and carried the corpses of their loved ones through the streets of New York. By the end of 1990, over 120,000 people in the United States had died of AIDS; a year later, a million Americans and nearly 10 million people worldwide had HIV.[21] It would be six years before life-saving combination therapies were made available to some people living with HIV; by then, over 362,000 people in the United States alone had died of AIDS.

Three decades after Queer Nation wrote their manifesto, I am sitting in my living room trying to conjure the sense of urgency it would take for me to get arrested or carry my dead through the streets in the name of queer and trans health. Anxiety blooms in my chest as I hunt for this feeling; it reminds me of frantically searching a purse or pocket for something important that isn't there. The truth is, I go to more meetings than protests these days, write more emails than manifestos.

The actions people took during the AIDS crisis were motivated by their experiences of massive death and collective grief and trauma in the face of violent government inaction. Queer and trans people and their allies channelled their love, grief, and rage into fighting back, and in the process changed systems and institutions. They put everything on the line because it was a matter of life or death. So much death.

My LGBTQ+ health work is motivated by a desire to keep queer and trans people alive in the face of conditions that harm or kill us. I, too, am driven by love, grief, and rage. Still, I sometimes fear I've been lulled into complacency. I notice where I've let the comfort of people who hold power in institutions like universities, medical schools, or hospitals diminish the force of my demands, and my condemnations. Some part of me believed if I asked nicely and didn't ask for more than they could give without ceding power, control, or resources, they would care enough to keep us alive. How often was I wrong? At what cost to my community?

Many of us who work in the field of queer and trans health are also members of the LGBTQ+ community. We live and work in contexts that try to force us to conform and hide the parts of ourselves deemed too unruly, too abnormal, too pathological, too perverted. This conformity becomes both a survival strategy and a means of gaining access to the systems and institutions we are trying to change. Yet as Alisa Bierria wrote on behalf of radical antiviolence organization Communities Against Rape and Abuse (CARA), "The dissonance of maintaining a real identity and a disguised one creates significant amounts of stress and consumes considerable amounts of precious time and resources that should be spent organizing."[22]

"Assimilate" is a verb; it suggests an active process. Action takes energy.

I am learning to remember that "pervert" is a verb, too.

Its origins are in Old French and Latin words meaning to undo, destroy, and subvert; to turn, transform, be changed. To pervert something is to alter its course, meaning, or state to distort or corrupt what was originally intended. It's often used in the negative ("to pervert the course of justice"), but if the system you are trying to change is fundamentally rooted in oppression, should it not be perverted?

Disabled Puerto Rican Jewish writer and activist Aurora Levins Morales writes, "It's worth discovering who your political ancestors are, tracing your genealogies of empowerment."[23] Today, when I look into that small gold mirror on my altar, I see my face reflected back to me and it reminds me who I am, where I come from, and who I'm accountable to. I feel a kinship with the generations of queer and trans ancestors who loved, fucked, and fought their way toward more liberated futures. I make a practice of thanking those ancestors. I promise to live and work in ways that will offer similar gifts to our descendants.

I promise to pervert the system.

It's no coincidence that queer perverts taught me how to take a punch—and how to throw one, how to achieve deep and precise impact without inadvertently damaging the delicate, breakable places you want to avoid. And the truth is, I want to pummel the systems and institutions killing the queer and trans people I love. I want to punch them into an entirely different shape or make them disappear altogether so we can grow something new in their place.

I want to pervert these systems and institutions, to let forth with the full force of the love, grief, and rage that propel me in this work.

I want to stop pulling my punches.

GIVE ME QUEER ALCHEMY

I once described myself in an interview as "a Trojan horse of radical values."[24] When audiences of health care providers, medical students, or academics look at me, they probably see a middle-aged white cis woman with a PhD whose work is grounded in the kinds of evidence you find in academic journals and textbooks. I'm most likely wearing a fashionable-yet-professional dress, lipstick, and high heels. I am legible to them as an expert in ways they are familiar with. In this way I am palatable: acceptable, agreeable, pleasant.

I keep picturing a bowl of vanilla pudding: soft, sweet, easy to swallow.

Then I imagine myself throwing the bowl of pudding at the wall, an explosion of sharp edges and messy spatters. I want a new container, something expansive and shape-shifting that feels good when I hold it in my hands. I want to fill it with salt water charged under a full moon, fragrant herbs and flowers, rocks from the ocean. I want to fill it with blood, piss, tears, and cum. I want to set it on fire. I want to mix the ashes into the earth and sink my hands into the soil up to my wrists. I want a spell of transformation.

Give me queer alchemy.

There's an undercurrent of queerness running through the definition of alchemy: "1. a power or process that changes or transforms something in a mysterious or impressive way; 2. an inexplicable or mysterious transmuting."[25] Queer and trans people are alchemists. We are mysterious, impressive, inexplicable, and powerful. We are skilled in the art of transformation.

In an essay called "Dream beyond the Wounds," adrienne maree brown writes: "Find the wounded places in your community, where thinking and action are stagnant—bring the medicine of imagination."[26] Queer and trans people are experts in the medicine of imagination. It is a form of expertise that has ensured our community's survival across generations yet is rarely recognized as such in medical, educational, or other institutional settings.

In these settings, LGBTQ+ health is frequently framed in terms of disparities, pathology, risk. Queer and trans people are a "vulnerable population." In more progressive spaces, our suffering is contextualized—minority stress, health inequities—but there often seems to be an undercurrent of otherness, shame and blame thrumming beneath the surface. We are sicker because of who and what we are and what we do, or don't do. I can picture an authoritative finger wagging at me, at us. In my mind's eye, this finger is attached to a stern older white man wearing a white coat and stethoscope, though the hard truth is that even the most progressive and well-intentioned among us can be complicit in this, and we often are.

I want queer alchemy because I want something more expansive, imaginative, and transformative than LGBTQ+ health care that is affirming or seeks to foster our resilience. Don't get me wrong, these things are important, but they are insufficient to transform the conditions of our lives. Having more tick boxes to choose from on a hospital admission form will not set us free. Dignified health care is vital to our well-being, but it shouldn't be our ultimate goal. I want us to dream bigger than this and demand more from the health system and the people whose job it is to care for us.

I've noticed that "resilience" is a word that gets tossed around a lot in conversations about LGBTQ+ health. It often seems to be conceptualized as a resource to be developed and extracted from us: people want to foster our resilience, promote it, understand where it comes from and how to create more of it. Trans and intersex scholar Hil Malatino offers a definition of resilience that feels both more accurate and much queerer to me: "Resilience is thus not about bouncing back, nor about moving forward, but rather a communal alchemical mutation of pain into possibility."[27]

Malatino gives us a different way of understanding resilience, a conceptualization that is more alchemical than extractive. It is an honouring of our brilliance, not a consolation prize for our suffering. Queer and trans communities have long histories of mutual aid because the circumstances of our lives—and our deaths—demand it of us. We understand that resilience isn't an individual property; it's shared and interactional.[28] As Malatino so astutely observes, we know how to move together to turn pain into possibility. We innovate to survive. We expect more than we are given, then we alchemize our dreams and desires into being.

I learned queer alchemy through my body. I've always bruised easily, patches of indigo blooming as blood vessels break under the surface of my pale skin. I carry those marks with me for days and weeks. I used to think of it as a painful inconvenience, my flaws visible to others. Being a queer pervert taught me to love my bruises, showed me how this quality of being easily marked can be delightful to my lovers and me. I am choosing the pain, not because I must endure it to survive but because it gives me pleasure and, at its best, can be a site of healing, discovery, and transformation. A threshold, a portal. Alchemy.

WHAT IT MEANS TO LEAVE NO ONE BEHIND

Disability justice–based performance project Sins Invalid asserts, "We are powerful not despite the complexities of our bodies, but because of them. We move together, with no body left behind."[29] Sins Invalid was cofounded in 2006 by Black disabled poet, activist, and author Leroy Moore and Patty Berne, a Japanese-Haitian queer disabled woman who now leads the organization. The idea of leaving no one behind is foundational to disability justice, a framework and practice rooted in the expertise and leadership of disabled people of colour and queer and gender diverse disabled people. Disability justice movements have rallied under the umbrella that no one is disposable; they understand we are all "beloved, kindred, needed."[30] As disabled queer scholar-activist Liat Ben-Moshe reminds us, "To do the work of liberation means to leave no one behind."[31]

Several years ago, I committed to learning more about disability justice. I've read and listened to the work and expertise of disabled people of colour and queer and gender diverse disabled people and I am beginning to practise what disability justice looks like in my life.

This shows up in practical ways, like going fragrance-free because it helps create access for others or learning how to cut ableist language out of my vocabulary. It also shows up more foundationally, like deepening into interdependence in my relationships and being more attentive to the needs and capacity of my body and those of the people around me. I am still so new in this learning process, yet what I have learned so far about disability justice has fundamentally changed how I understand health and healing, how I relate to my own and other people's body/minds, and how I show up in the world. It has vastly expanded and shifted my sense of possibilities for what health care and mutual aid can look like.

This acknowledgment feels important because it was through a conversation with Leah Lakshmi Piepzna-Samarasinha, a queer disabled autistic nonbinary Sri Lankan/Roma/Irish femme writer and disability/transformative justice worker, that I realized how deeply I've internalized the idea that it is necessary to leave people—and parts of myself—behind in order to create a health system better able to meet the needs of LGBTQ+ people. My radical politics were no match for the ways ableism, individualism, respectability politics, white supremacy, and homonormativity have wormed their way under my skin.

I'm coming to understand how the belief *someone* must always be left behind has infiltrated, shaped, and limited my conceptualization of queer and trans health and healing. Has it infiltrated and limited yours, too? I invite you to think about how you've learned to leave parts of yourself or your community behind to access health care because you know it's unsafe or impossible to get care when you show up in the fullness and complexity of who you are.

We learn to leave behind parts of ourselves and our communities as the price of gaining access to institutions and systems designed according to norms and assumptions we'll never fit into, whether we're accessing those spaces as patient, provider, student, educator, advocate, or activist. As we do the work of systemic change, it's imperative we remember these systems weren't made for us or by us and in some cases were created to discipline, control, or eradicate us and our queer and trans kin.

Too often, queer and trans people seeking to access health care are required to apply a veneer of "normalcy" and "respectability" to our lives and bodies to achieve a form of conditional acceptance inside a system that wasn't designed for us. We rarely if ever show our whole selves to our health care providers; we are practiced at the tactics and survival strategies of concealment and elision. I'm thinking of all the times I've left out the details of who and how I fuck, what brings me pleasure, who I count as family, which traumas I am willing to reveal. Like allopathic medicine, I break myself down into parts and try to be strategic about which ones will be held up to scrutiny.

Our health system often demands queer and trans people take the care we are given without complaint, even if it is violent, inadequate, or just plain wrong, often at great personal and/or financial cost. It gaslights us into disbelieving what we deeply know and understand to be true in our bodies. It pathologizes, shames, and blames us. It categorizes and ranks us in a hierarchy of worthiness that dictates how we are treated or if we are treated at all. Our health system excludes so many queer and trans people from receiving care, and it sometimes kills us or hastens our deaths.

This is not an individual experience. It is a collective one, the violent impacts of which are inequitably distributed across the LGBTQ+ community. What I mean by this is, we leave some people behind much more often. This is no accident. As is often the case in LGBTQ+ communities and mainstream movements, the people we leave behind are the ones who can't easily conform or assimilate to homonormative (white supremacist, ableist, capitalist) ideals of respectability. Queer and trans folks reading this, I'm asking us to reflect on how we are complicit in this abandonment. Yes, the health system leaves our people behind, and so do we.

When I think about who often gets left behind, I think of Black, Indigenous, and people of colour; trans, nonbinary, and gender diverse people—especially trans women of colour and transfeminine people; disabled, neurodiverse, and Mad people; fat people; and older people. I think about sex workers; people who use drugs; people who are homeless, underhoused, or street involved; poor people; migrants; and people who are currently or formerly incarcerated. I think about bisexual and pansexual people, asexual and aromantic people, people in kink and BDSM communities, polyamorous people, and people who have sex with multiple partners.

When I look at this list, I'm struck by how many of the queer and trans people I love fall into these categories, and how they bear the brunt of the health disparities that limit the life chances of people in the LGBTQ+ community. Who does the system classify as "healthy" and worthy of care? Who isn't classified this way, and why? Whose lives does the medical industrial complex deem as worth saving and whose lives are deemed disposable? The system is designed this way and it's our job to disrupt it, to pervert it. This, too, is a matter of life or death.

I keep returning to a question Audre Lorde asked in 1982: "Survival is not a theory. In what way do I contribute to the subjugation of any part of those who I define as my people?"[32] There is a gap between how I would answer her question today and what I want my answer to be; my work is to narrow that gap, a process that demands accountability, solidarity, and sustained effort. As Sins Invalid says, *"We move together, with no body left behind."* How might orienting to this phrase change our entire way of thinking about LGBTQ+ health and healing?

In asking this question, I'm not offering something new—rather, I'm pointing back and outward to lineages and contemporary practices of disability justice, mutual aid, interdependence, and community care. I'm challenging the exclusionary hierarchies and limiting constructions of expertise that characterize our health and medical education systems.

To leave no one behind is not just a moral and ethical imperative. It is a site of expansive possibilities. It is an invitation to dream into a vision of LGBTQ+ health and healing that far exceeds what we have been conditioned to accept.

BODIES OF KNOWLEDGE: I DIDN'T LEARN ABOUT QUEER AND TRANS HEALTH FROM A TEXTBOOK

Where did you learn about queer and trans health and healing? In asking this question, I don't mean learning that takes place in a classroom or lecture hall; I mean the kind of learning you do through your body and by being in relationship, through witnessing, listening, and generous sharing. What knowledge do you carry with you and take care to pass on? Who were your teachers and mentors? Who listened and helped you remember you were worthy of care? What teachings came to you like a gift, a balm, a lifeline? Who moved with you in a way that made sure you didn't get left behind?

I know this for sure: I didn't get this knowledge from doctors or pamphlets or public service announcements. You can't find it in textbooks or research articles in academic journals. I've never seen it in a PowerPoint presentation. The most important things I know about queer and trans health and healing I learned from my community and through my queer femme body.

My teachers were the femmes and drag queens who helped me understand there was a place for me in queerness and invited me into a community of writers, musicians, sex workers, filmmakers, artists, and activists inspired by the do-it-yourself (DIY) ethos of queer punk. Together, we created physical spaces of exuberant queer joy and radical self-expression that intentionally challenged binaries and oppressive norms. I learned about queer and trans health and healing on the dance floor, in a swirl of glitter and feathers, surrounded by a community of friends, lovers, and strangers. Once I started co-organizing queer dance parties with my friends, those dance floors also taught me important early lessons about collaboration, deescalation, harm reduction, antiracism, and what it takes to make events more accessible for disabled people.

Becoming part of a community of femmes offered me pathways to healing by showing me it was possible to be queer and feel like myself. Femmes taught me femininity could be queer as fuck (and in so doing, helped me avoid what would have been an awkward-for-me short hair and chain wallet phase in the early 2000s). Twenty years later, femmes still thrill and delight me with the myriad ways we embody and express our femininities. Femme is telling the stranger in front of you in the lineup for the gender-neutral washroom, "I love your lipstick!" and having them respond, "I love your earrings!" Femme community taught me what it's like to feel an immediate kinship with someone I just met.

Together with a group of five femme friends, I was part of a book club-turned-coven where we spent a year working our way through Barbara Carrellas's book *Ecstasy Is Necessary*. It was deeply potent healing work that culminated in a weekend-long ecstatic retreat facilitated by our friend the trans witch somatic sex educator. Femmes taught me about empowered sexuality, owning my power, and satiating my desires. Femmes showed me how to love fiercely, with an open heart and sturdy boundaries. Femmes taught me how to put on my armour, how to make it beautiful, and when to take it off. Femmes were there for me every time I fell apart. Femme is an ethic of care.

Queer perverts and leatherdykes have taught me many lessons, both profane and practical, about health, healing, and what it means to show up for your people. Ready for anything, they know how to band together and get shit done. Queer perverts and leatherdykes are ingenious, highly skilled, and wildly, often diabolically, creative. This is who I want to be with when the apocalypse hits. They know how to stay calm under pressure and will just happen to have on hand an array of tools, rope, a knife, a well-stocked first aid kit, allergy-safe snacks, and some bottled water. I learned about queer and trans health and healing in dungeons, play parties, workshops, hotel rooms, and bedrooms, bearing witness to and participating in the countless ways we embody our desires. Queer perverts and leatherdykes understand there are many paths to healing and there is power in choosing your trials. As queer femme educators and trauma survivors Masti Khor and Chanelle Gallant write in the *Kink and Trauma* zine, "Consensual BDSM puts us in situations where our bodies feel distressed, but this time we have control over the situation and our bodies. This can be incredibly healing."[33] The containers we create together can be a crucible and it is a sacred gift to hold each other as we challenge our edges.

It was queer perverts and leatherdykes who helped me understand consent as an ongoing, embodied, collaborative process that feels more like a dance than a transaction. They showed me what it looks and feels like to be trauma-informed by demonstrating an adept awareness of how our past experiences can show up in our bodies and interactions with each other. We can't make our past traumas go away, but we can learn to hold them and each other more skilfully, and we can heal together. Queer perverts and leatherdykes invited me into a continuous process of discovering new facets of myself and naming my desires, no matter how weird or shameful those desires might feel. They showed me what it looks like to be generous in sharing your knowledge, expansive in your definitions of family, and proud of your identity as a sexual outlaw.

I know how to leave, but it was the queer community who taught me how to stay. Part of me is always primed to flee, a trauma response that has kept me safe but isn't the one-size-fits-every-situation tool my nervous system sometimes tells me it is. The experience of living in the same city for twenty years and fostering a queer community there has taught me how to put down roots, build community, and nuture and tend relationships; in this way, it's offered me important lessons about health and healing as contextual, collective processes. When I moved to Vancouver in 2001, I hadn't even come out to myself yet. I moved west for graduate school, not expecting to find an identity, a community, and a chosen family in the process. Back then, I was twenty-two and accustomed to a particular kind of transience, moving apartments every year and periodically uprooting myself (or, when I was a kid, being uprooted) to move to an entirely new city. I hadn't yet learned to stay or that family could be bigger than the tight circle of my mom and me.

Queer and trans people taught me what it means to put down roots and how to invest in a community. They showed me how staying in one place can be a brave and loving act. All kinds of relationships—friendship, romantic, and sexual—have formed, fractured, been repaired, and stayed broken over the past two decades of my life in Vancouver's LGBTQ+ community. We are intimate with the details of each other's lives and histories because we share a physical place, a geographic and social proximity that sometimes feels suffocating and often feels wonderful. Being part of this community has helped me understand, create, and deepen into chosen family.

This experience has taught me that the work of accountability and repair moves at its own pace, often slowly. It has shown me how boundary setting is an embodied process that's as much about an enthusiastic "Yes!" or a confident "Not right now" than it is about a definitive "No." It also taught me that "No" is a full sentence. This community is where I've done my earliest, most important, and ongoing learning about antiracism, disability justice, and what it means to commit to allyship, solidarity, and collective liberation as lifelong practices. The queer and trans community I'm part of has taught me about mutual aid and creating what we need because no one else is going to do it for us. I learned about queer and trans health and healing at potlucks, protests, house parties, fundraisers, rituals, kitchens, coffee shops, parks, and all the other spaces where I've gathered with my community for the past two decades.

QUEER AND TRANS HEALTH AND HEALING IS INFINITE

I carry the knowledge I've learned about health and healing from all of these people, communities, experiences, and places in my body. Here's some of what I know.

Queer and trans health and healing is sacred and profane

It is magic, altars, and do-it-yourself rituals. It is intimacy with death and grief; it can be a haunting. It is knowing who your queer and trans ancestors are and honouring them. *What is remembered, lives.* It is dungeons and alleys, bathhouses, and parks. Queer and trans health and healing is figuring out how to fuck and experience pleasure more safely during this pandemic and the next one, and sharing what you learn so other people can do it, too. It's being so skilled at this that glory holes even make their way into official public health guidelines. It's knowing exactly what size of latex or nitrile glove you wear. It's revelling in the pleasure of your own touch or spooning with your best friend. Queer and trans health and healing is embodied. It is erotic. It is wild. It will gush out of you like a river or drip slowly, transfixing. It has knives, fists, and fangs. It will hold the softest parts of you with more tenderness than you imagined possible.

Queer and trans health and healing
is fucking up, learning how to be better,
trying and sometimes failing

It's practising what it looks like to live accountably and figuring out how to have boundaries in a context of interdependence. It's being best friends with your exes or never talking to them again. I don't think it's a coincidence that a lot of queer and trans folks—especially those who are Black, Indigenous, and people of colour and/or disabled—are leaders and teachers in movements for transformative justice and police and prison abolition. Queer and trans health and healing is designing creative, community-led strategies for intervening on and preventing violence. It's understanding and practising consent as an ongoing embodied dialogue. It's holding each other's trauma and our own and learning through our bodies how much of each we can sustainably carry and what we want to let go of. It's someone saying, "I believe you" and meaning it.

Queer and trans health and healing
is do-it-yourself and do-it-together

It's sharing knowledge and information that doesn't exist in medical textbooks, clinics, or doctors' offices about how to honour and care for ourselves, our identities, and our bodies. We make it up as we go along while drawing on generations of wisdom passed down from community elders who might be younger than us. It's wedging ourselves into the cracks in the system and expertly traversing our way around rigid binaries and boxes that seek to limit who we are and how we love. Queer and trans health and healing is delivering meals after someone has gender-affirming surgery and donating to crowdfunding campaigns. It's being skilled at mutual aid because we've learned to not trust the state to take care of us. Queer and trans health and healing is sharing food and making tinctures. It's caring for children and older people with curiosity, humility, generosity, patience, and love. It's caring for caregivers the same way. It's caring for each other. It's caring for ourselves.

Queer and trans health and healing
is disability justice

Disability justice understands that "all bodies are unique and essential" with "strengths and needs that must be met."[34] It reminds us our power derives from the complexities of our bodies, not despite them, and that our bodies are inseparable from our intersecting identities and contexts. Queer and trans health and healing is a legacy of resistance, creativity, innovation, and valuing body/minds in all their shapes and manifestations. It's swapping meds and dropping off soup and passing on strategies for living with chronic illness or disability. It's access check-ins, ramps, fragrance-free events, sign language interpretation, and crip time. It's fighting to change ableist laws and policies. It's doing everything you can to keep someone alive or out of an institution and sometimes succeeding. Queer and trans health and healing is an ongoing practice of interdependence, when it's easy and especially when it's hard.

Queer and trans health and healing
is reducing harm today while transforming
the system for the future

It's being pen pals with a queer or trans person who's locked up and helping them access housing, income, community, and any other supports they need when they're released. Queer and trans health and healing is learning how to help someone in crisis or deescalate a conflict so nobody calls 911. It's never seeing another cop in a pride parade again because we abolished the police. It's fighting for prison abolition and the abolition of all carceral spaces. Queer and trans health and healing is carrying naloxone and fighting for the decriminalization of drugs. It's contributing to your local sex worker–led organization, walking or rolling in the annual Red Umbrella march and supporting the decriminalization of sex work. It's fighting for housing for all, a world without borders, and saying, "Yes in my backyard." If you're a settler like me, queer and trans health and healing is understanding it never was your backyard, anyway. It's learning whose land you're on and supporting Indigenous land defenders.

Queer and trans health and healing is knowing that activism happens in bedrooms, kitchens, meeting rooms, on the internet, in psych wards, jails, doctors' offices, play parties, overdose prevention sites, forests, gardens, massage parlours, on stages, in classrooms, bookstores, via text message, and in every other place you can imagine. It's coming up with strategies to help you or someone you love survive another minute, hour, day, or year.

Queer and trans health and healing is knowing that, in spite of all the systems that try to kill us, we are worthy of being alive, we are loved, and there are ways for us to exist joyfully in the fullest expressions of who we are.

REMEMBER: WE WILL GET OUR ASSES KICKED, AND WE WILL WIN

To be queer and trans is to be an alchemist, a transformation artist, a world builder, a survivor of conditions that would rather have you dead. It is to be intimate with a potent mix of love, grief, and rage. To be queer and trans is to know how to stay inside the pain and alchemize it into the medicine of imagination.

When I feel hopeless about the future, as I sometimes do, I remember our community's ability to survive across generations and the lineage of ancestors who are with us now, bringing their own medicine of imagination. Thirty years ago, the Queer Nation manifesto told us there are "two important things to remember about the coming revolutions. The first is that we will get our asses kicked. The second is that we will win." May we always remember this. May we move together in a way that leaves no one behind.

Pleasure as the Baseline

Interview with Dawn Serra

Dawn Serra is a therapeutic sex and relationship coach and pleasure advocate based in Vancouver, BC. Her work as a white cis middle-class queer fat survivor is a fiercely compassionate invitation for each of us to deepen our relationships with our bodies and our pleasure as an antidote to the trauma, disconnection, and isolation so many of us feel. Our conversation grew out of our shared interest in exploring the idea of what pleasure-centred health care could look like for LGBTQ+ people.

Zena: What does pleasure mean to you?

Dawn: At a basic level, pleasure is about aliveness. It's the part of us that makes us feel connected to something. It's a way for us to be in our bodies. Pleasure only ever exists in the now. It requires us to arrive and is an opportunity to feel into the edges of what it means to be us. No one else can experience pleasure in this body. No one else knows what it's like to feel these sensations. Pleasure is the ultimate experience of owning and arriving in this body and this life.

Zena: It seems like we often associate pleasure with sex or the erotic. How do you understand the connections between pleasure, sexuality, and the erotic, and how are they distinct from each other?

Dawn: I see sex as a small piece of something much larger, which we would categorize as the erotic. The erotic is part of what it means to experience pleasure. The erotic, the life force, and the creative energy Audre Lorde talks about in her 1978 essay "Uses of the Erotic: The Erotic as Power," is a huge part of pleasure. But it's not the only inroad.

When we think about pleasure, we often think of something special, something tied to big events, important moments, or the need to escape our lives. Pleasure isn't only cake on your birthday or fancy meals at holidays. One of the things that helps people when they're grappling with what it means to heal is to find ways to experience pleasure in the everyday. It's finding the smallest moments in our lives that help us arrive and feeling into them. It's waiting to see what reveals itself that gives you a moment of "Yes!" For me, pleasure is colours that bring me joy. It's flavours. It's smells. It's touches from humans and nonhumans. Pleasure is another way of truly being with the sensations, questions, and opportunities our bodies are offering us.

Zena: How do you see the connections between pleasure and health, in general and specifically for queer and trans folks?

Dawn: One of the things I think about a lot when it comes to pleasure and health is how white supremacy, racism, colonialism, capitalism, and ableism keep all of us feeling disconnected and over-whelmed. It's this feeling of "Well, I will do this thing that makes me feel good when this injury is healed, or when I've changed my body size to be bigger or smaller, or when I make a certain amount of money." There's an aspirational aspect to it, an "I'll deserve it when ..." We've internalized dominant cultural stories dictating who's deserving. Often, if our experience of health isn't aligned with what's marketed as the ideal, or if we're struggling with something like chronic pain, dysphoria, or trauma, pleasure becomes framed as something we'll get to when these other things are resolved. I would love so much for us to be able to feel more worthy of pleasure no matter what we're experiencing, no matter what our level of health is.

I'm also interested in how we can bring pleasure into places that have historically been painful. For so many people, especially trans, nonbinary, and queer folks, as well as Black, Indigenous, and people of colour, fat folks, disabled folks, and other people who experience marginalization, asking for help has led to policing, institutionalization, rejection of resources, loss of access, and harm. When I think about pleasure and health, I think about more opportunities for vitality and arriving exactly as we are, regardless of what we're going through and how our body looks, and also being able to experience more support and validation when we do ask for help.

So often the bar in health care is to eliminate pain. I understand the importance of this—pain is debilitating for many people, and our health system isn't well equipped to care for people who experience chronic pain. At the same time, I'm interested in growing our capacity to ask questions that position pleasure as the baseline. Pleasure is often treated as a nice-to-have when, really, it's essential. It's crucial. It's what makes this life something we want to continue showing up for.

Zena: How do you understand the connections between pleasure and liberation? How can pleasure help queer and trans folks get free?

Dawn: Pleasure is literally the experience of *your* body, so it becomes really complicated when you don't feel like your body is yours or when the people around you don't understand your body, or they want to control it. Pleasure is getting to decide what happens to these vessels we're inside of. It's living life on our own terms. I get to decide what feels good today and it might be different from yesterday or tomorrow. No one could possibly know this except for me because I'm the only one in my body.

Liberation is about choice, power, and sovereignty. Pleasure is the ultimate expression of that. Related questions I've been exploring are: Who gets to have ownership of their body? Who gets to decide what happens to their body, and when? Pleasure can happen in big and small ways, but we need a baseline of safety first. Emily Nagoski's TED talk taught me that our brains can't code something as pleasurable without a relative amount of safety, and for many of us the circumstances of our lives make it difficult to feel safe. To feel pleasure, we need a feeling of relative safety—not total safety, but enough to feel good and be able to ask ourselves, "What is making me thrive? What is bringing me joy? How do I want to show up?" Pleasure invites those questions, and there's so much creativity in that.

Zena: If you had the power to design pleasure-centred health care, what would it look and feel like?

Dawn: One of the first things I think about is the physical design of the space. Are there comfortable chairs that fit my fat body? Are there colours that feel wonderful to me? I think about the sensory experience of the fabrics, smells, colours, lighting, and art. What are the spaces we just love being in, and why can't our health care spaces be those places? Why can't we feel a sense of exhalation when we arrive because it feels good to be there and we know we're going to be supported and seen?

I also think about my relationships with the people who care for me. Can we truly be in relationship with each other, not in a hierarchy or a power struggle? Can we come from a place of respect, responsibility, and recognition of each other's humanity? Can we share knowledge and collaborate? I want my health care providers to know who's in my life and what's important to me. I want to know about my health care provider and how they're existing in the community, so we have an opportunity to cocreate experiences that serve my life and my body. I want to be able to tell them the scary truths or ask the difficult questions and know that no matter what, I'm going to be witnessed, and together, we can decide if we want to work on it or not because we have a reciprocal, meaningful relationship.

Zena: What do you think health care providers would need to learn as part of their training to become pleasure-centred? What would your curriculum look like?

Dawn: I'd start with helping them learn their own experiences of body and pleasure. If someone wants to go into a profession that helps facilitate spaces for healing, they need to start with themself. What are your experiences of boundaries and consent? Do you understand your body and your edges and how to communicate around them? Where do you notice things feeling tender and shameful and scary? I want health care providers' training to be about empathy and understanding the role of pleasure in their lives, and the barriers to it, so they become more skilful at talking about pleasure with patients, including when people are experiencing pain or are in crisis. I think it's important for providers to normalize conversations where we can talk about what feels good.

I would love to have health care providers ask me questions like: What brings you a greater sense of aliveness? How might we work with your body to find ways to make the things you enjoy doing feel more ease filled? What kinds of support would help you to experience less burnout? What kinds of pleasure are you experiencing? What can we do that increases your pleasure or gets you to a place where pleasure becomes possible? Questions like these open up different conversations and create opportunities to dream, create, and share resources.

Becoming pleasure-centred also necessitates attention to health care providers' learning and working conditions. What kinds of support do they have? What kind of power exists in their schooling and learning? What kind of accessibility do they have? I imagine this radical future where those of us seeking care feel utterly supported and like we have lots of choice and the people providing care feel extraordinarily supported and able to be vulnerable. I think this would help our care providers' way of working and learning feel more generative and less about burnout, tolerating, pushing through, and performing a certain level of wellness.

It would also make it easier for Black, Indigenous, and people of colour, disabled people, sex workers, queer and trans people, fat people, parents, and others who don't fit the narrow stereotype of what a health care provider looks like to become health care providers. When it's not about working a forty-eight-hour shift with three hours of sleep or getting through a hundred patients in a week, people with radically different identities, experiences, and abilities can provide health care, too. If health care providers were brought up inside of a system where collaboration was deeply valued over competitiveness or being able to outlast or outperform, I think it would help enable people to show up with more curiosity, empathy, and a commitment to finding our way together.

Zena: Have you experienced health care that has felt pleasurable? And if yes, how did it feel and what did it look like? What was happening in your body?

Dawn: I've had small moments that have been incredibly meaningful, but it's not enough to stitch together a quilt. I was doing community acupuncture for a while and one of the things I loved about it was seeing people that I knew, sharing space with them, being treated openly with other people, and being able to get hugs from friends and check in with each other.

I've had an incredible experience with my therapist. Instead of focusing on my trauma and pain, of which I have plenty, we focus on continually orienting back toward the things that make me feel good, the things that feel easy and pleasurable. One hundred percent of the work we do is about continually reorienting in that direction because it's so easy for me, and I know I'm not alone in this, to get pulled into the things that feel scary, to focus on all the things I'm avoiding, and then to feel bad about that. Our work is a gentle, beautiful reminder to orient toward what's possible. I've never been in relationship with a health care provider whose primary goal was to help me find more entry points into presence, ease, and pleasure.

Zena: What does that reorientation look and feel like in practice?

Dawn: This has been an ongoing learning curve for me because I exist inside of white supremacy and capitalism, so I have this urge to be like, "Okay, I'm supposed to be orienting toward pleasure, so I'm going to do that every day for at least five minutes or I'm going to look for ten ways I can do the thing." Check mark, check mark, check mark! Lists, lists, lists! Do the things! And then when I don't, I'm going to feel guilty about it.

Zena: [*laughing*] I feel so called out right now!

Dawn: I know! So part of my work has been to just name this over and over again. It's been a practice where, if I go two weeks between sessions and my takeaway was to notice all the places on my body where I feel ease every day, and I only did it one time for ten seconds, what a win! That is literally what my therapist and I then celebrate as a win. She'll ask, "How did those ten seconds feel? Let's explore it; let's stretch into it." It's a process of asking the question and being inside of it for a little while, really feeling into it and asking, "What does this mean for me?" And then trusting that because I've got that question inside of me, I'm going to start having little moments of pleasure or curiosity that gently start revealing themselves.

It's very slow, which is also really agitating, you know? But over the course of many months, I'll start noticing that it's easier for me to feel into the places in my body that aren't in pain while pain is happening, and that I'm having lots of little moments of gently letting the question unfold rather than pushing toward forcing any answer. Every single time, my therapist helps me find new ways to hold those questions, which means my tool box and my skills become more developed through this very gentle unfolding.

Even though it's so tempting to answer your question with something specific, it's actually been more about the relationship with my therapist, where I feel like I can't fail and I'm not going to get it wrong. That makes it okay for it to be slow and awkward and for me to not do it all the time. It's a matter of gently returning over and over; like anyone on a meditation cushion says, by doing these small returns to self over time, radical changes become possible.

Zena: There's a liberatory quality to what you're describing.

Dawn: Yeah. Because one of the things that has been such a barrier for me personally, and I know I'm not alone, is only accessing health care when things are bad enough. Which is to say when things are *really* bad. When I'm really suffering, when I just can't drag myself out of bed anymore because my sickness or pain has gotten intolerable, then I try and get some type of treatment.

My relationship with my therapist is different in that we're collaboratively exploring and building something together so that when I experience a crisis or something is really hard, we have a rich history and foundation we can trust. I wish I had this kind of relationship with all my health care providers. If I can be in relationship with you throughout my life, we're going to notice things much sooner and discover so much more potential pleasure than if I wait until things have become intolerable, which might cause me additional harm.

Zena: What are some concrete strategies that individual health care providers could use to make their queer and trans patients' experiences of accessing health care more pleasurable?

Dawn: The first thing that comes to mind for me is cultivating curiosity. Instead of trying to get everyone to fit some arbitrary standard or whatever you categorize as "normal," enter each room with curiosity, even if it means an extra few minutes' worth of questions like, "What would a win feel like for you? What would 'better' feel like for you? What would help you feel respected and seen?" Being able to ask questions like this allows people to share their humanity and their uniqueness.

The other thing I think would be helpful is for providers to take an inventory of the spaces where they practise. Do chairs have arms so that people in bigger bodies are uncomfortable when they sit in them? Is the lighting you're using making people feel especially exposed and vulnerable? Those might not be things you can change right away, but acknowledging them can make a difference: "I'm sorry these chairs are uncomfortable; we're working on it" or "I recognize these lights kind of make you feel like you're in a spotlight." Being able to name that you notice these things, even if you don't have the capacity to immediately change them, helps signal to someone that you care about them and are thinking about their experience.

Zena: How can we seek out and create pleasure in our everyday lives?

Dawn: At a very basic level, one of the things we all have to start with, which is hard for so many of us, is believing our pleasure matters. Do we feel worthy of pleasure, which also means owning our hungers and desires? If we fundamentally believe that pleasure is a human right, it starts to shift the conversation. And if experiencing pleasure feels scary or threatening, it could help to begin with getting support around this.

Pleasure asks us to arrive in our body, in the moment, so it's important to consider how safe we feel to do this, in big and small ways. To arrive in our bodies and to feel more alive is one of the most sacred experiences we can have as human beings. Can I enjoy this meal, be with this food, think about where it came from, and share it with people I care about? Can I appreciate these colours and smells? This requires us to start feeling. Something that's so complicated about this is, if we're going to start centring pleasure, we're also opening ourselves up to deeper grief, to deeper sadness, and to feeling more deeply in all areas of our life. We need to have more support and community that helps us to access pleasure and celebrate the nuance and the complexity of it.

Zena: If you were to invite readers to do an experiment with pleasure, what could that experiment look like?

Dawn: There's a prescriptive "just do it!" mentality around pleasure that I find really challenging. People who live in more normative bodies often say, "It's easy, just do it, pleasure feels good, always go for the orgasm!" But when we've experienced trauma and pain, leaving our body is a wise and powerful survival technique. Returning to the body can be terrifying. In order to do an experiment with pleasure, we need to begin by noticing what helps us feel safe enough to arrive and to feel.

For some people a safe place to start might be looking for a colour that brings you pleasure. Maybe it's blue, so you can do an experiment by asking, "Where can I start noticing blues?" When you notice blue, pause for just a moment to delight in each blue. That can be an extraordinary pleasure experiment because each time you notice blue, you're arriving in that moment and then, if you need to, you can leave again. It's very gentle and accessible. You can do similar experiments with touch. How many things can you touch to discover which textures bring you pleasure? It's playful and silly, but it's also a way for us to arrive without forcing ourselves to do something that might not feel safe or available to us.

I always want to start with the smallest thing that I can do while still feeling safe. For me, that usually means coming back to the senses. A flavour, a colour, a sound, a smell, a touch, and then I build on that experiment. If you do these kinds of experiments, I find that after a while you start noticing how many inroads there are to arriving in this body of yours.

All those small things start to open us to bigger and bigger things. I would encourage people to start with this practice and see what it reveals. You might be really surprised at what you find.

There may be some people—and, certainly, depending on the day, I would be one of them—for whom thinking about pleasure in health care experiences feels terrifying and dangerous. I want to name that if that's true, it's true for a very good reason. It's probably been really dangerous in a number of ways for you to interact with health care providers.

If that's true, can we hold that while still asking: Do I feel deserving of pleasure and what would help bring more pleasure into my life? Being able to carry that knowledge with us into health care settings, even if we don't articulate it, can bring us a new sense of power and help move us toward greater freedom and liberation.

Cripping Healing

Leah Lakshmi Piepzna-Samarasinha

Dedicated to Lucia Leandro "LL" Gimeno,
May 3, 1979–April 19, 2021. #LLForever

What if your body/mind has never and will never fit into the western medical industrial complex's definition of "health"?

What if there is no "cure" for what ails you? (i.e., your disability, Deafness, neurodivergence*, chronic illness)

What if you don't want to be cured? But you might want an individual thing mended?

What if you know that the cures that are offered to us often kill us?

What does "healing" mean to you/us?

One of the foundational beliefs of most health care systems is that there's one definition of health, everyone wants it, and it's been the same forever. Health is like puppies and babies and blue skies— unquestionably, uncomplicatedly good.

---

*   The terms "neurodivergent" and "neurodivergence" were created by a multiply neurodivergent Hapa (biracial Asian) long-time autistic activist and writer Kassiane Asasumasu, to refer to the state of having a brain, nervous system, or both that operates different from the typical. Neurodivergence is a broad framework that encompasses everything from autism to ADHD, multiplicity/plurality, schizophrenia, traumatic brain injury, cerebral palsy, dementia, and more. For more on this, see Dani Alexis, "What Is Neurodivergence?," January 9, 2021, https://danialexis .net/2020/01/09/what-is-neurodivergence/ and check out the blog *Radical Neurodivergence Speaking* (http://timetolisten.blogspot.com).

Healing means fixing. A wound, a burn, cancer: no one wants those things. I'm not opposed to this idea. I like my cuts stitched up and my tumours taken away, too. But in the overarching medical industrial complex (MIC) definition of the term, healing also means fixing the disabled, Deaf, neurodivergent body/mind into a normal abled, sane one. Because, in their minds, no one would want to be those things.

People can deal with deconstructing a lot of things. But try saying that not everyone wants to be cured or healthy or can be*, that "health" is subjective and there's no one universal definition of it, and that the current definition of what health is is just an idea that somebody made up (or, in the words of the Dude from *The Big Lebowski*, "Yeah, well, that's just your opinion, man") and people will look at you like you have three heads.

However, disabled Cherokee Two-Spirit scholar Qwo-Li Driskill reminds us, "Ableism is colonial. It is employed to maintain an ideal body of a white supremacist imagination. The ideal body is heterosexual, male, white, Christian, non-disabled, and well-muscled. It is an ideal with a long and troubling history inseparable from racism, genocide, misogyny, and eugenics."[35]

That ideal white abled cis male Christian thin body is the same "healthy" body the MIC holds over our heads. To them, every other kind of body and mind is a flaw to be fixed, a broken toy. In the MIC's world view, there have never been times before settler colonialism when fat bodies were seen as desirable and healthy or cultures where

---

* Health is also increasingly seen as a moral imperative. Health at Every Size® doctor Fall Ferguson defines healthism as "the often unspoken idea that there is a moral value to health; it emerges as the assumption that people *should* pursue health. It's the contempt in the non-smoker's attitude toward smokers; it's the ubiquitous sneer against couch potatoes. Healthism includes the idea that anyone who isn't healthy just isn't trying hard enough or has some moral failing or sin to account for." See Fall Ferguson, "The HAES® Files: Speculations on Healthism & Privilege," Association for Size Diversity and Health, November 19, 2013, https://healthateverysizeblog.org/2013/11/19/the-haes-files-speculations-on-healthism-privilege/.

Deafness or bipolarity or autism or being a little person weren't seen as defects, but ordinary ways to be human. But health has been defined differently in every culture throughout history, and that definition is always political.

In stark contrast, a foundational disability justice (a movement created by disabled Black, Indigenous, and people of colour and/ or queer and trans people in 2005, centring our visions, needs, and demands as disabled QT/BPOC) idea is that there is no one right or wrong way to have a body. Disability justice believes that disabled body/minds are a regular part of the continuum of being human— that there have always been disabled, neurodivergent, chronically ill, Deaf, and Blind people since there have been people. Before ableist settler colonialism, there were a million ways to have a body or a mind and none of those were automatically wrong.*

Aurora Levins Morales and Patty Berne, two of the BIPOC queer women who are foundational activist creators of the disability justice movement, wrote,

> All bodies are unique and essential.
> All bodies are whole.
> All bodies have strengths and needs that must be met.
> We are powerful not despite the complexities of our bodies, but because of them.[36]

Let those revolutionary words sink in. How do they make you feel?

How does it change the way we imagine healing when there is no one "normal" "ideal" body/mind? No "normal" people with no access needs, and everyone else with "special" needs? But everyone having

---

* For more on this, see Sins Invalid's "10 Principles of Disability Justice": https://static1.square space.com/static/5bed3674f8370ad8c02efd9a/t/5f1f0783916d8a179c46126d/1595869064521/10_ Principles_of_DJ-2ndEd.pdf and the book *Skin, Tooth, and Bone: The Basis of Movement Is Our People*, 2nd ed. (Sins Invalid, 2019).

body/mind needs that will shift through our lifetimes—needs and bodily complexities that are not deficits, but hold power?

TOTALLY AWESOME SICK AND DISABLED LIVES

What healing do you need to thrive as a disabled, sick, Deaf, or neurodivergent person?

What's your own version of healing that doesn't have being fixed into abled or "normal" as an end goal?

What do you need to even start asking that question, and keep asking it?

These questions never get raised in medical school, most health care settings, or coffee break conversations about being sick, Mad, or disabled. We are not asked what our version of healing is. Yet, every sick, disabled, Mad, and neurodivergent person I've ever met has been able to easily tell me what they wanted and needed, and a ton of detailed information they knew about their body/mind, what hurt and what helped. It's just that most doctors never asked, or trusted their answers when they did ask.

The social model of disability—a way of understanding disability created by disabled activists in the United Kingdom in the 1980s, which says that the things that make disabled lives hard often aren't our disabled bodies or minds but an inaccessible world that actively tries to kill us, doesn't get taught to doctors and nurse practitioners and EMTs and massage therapists. The concepts of disabled skills, disabled people having communities, disabled ways of loving, befriending, supporting, the pride we have in ourselves as "disabled people knowing we are powerful and beautiful because of who we are, not despite it," as Stacey Park Milbern said, are concepts that are completely absent in health care settings and everyday life.[37] Yet all of these things are key ways we create wonderful, pleasurable, and powerful disabled lives. Crip community, relationships, mutual aid, and pride are core things that create high qualities of life. High qualities of life that are crip healing.

Crip is (certain) disabled community slang for being disabled. It works like the word "queer" does for queer people—a reclamation of a word that's been used against us. It's defiant, sly, a wink, or a head nod saying we see you rolling or limping or looking weird down the street, and we like what we see. Crip is a middle finger to the squeamish, bless-your-heart "tolerance" of terms like "differently abled."

Cripping is the verb form of the noun. We crip life when we bring beds to protests, centre our hangouts around the couch or one friend's accessible apartment, make a makeshift ramp by taking our sneakers off and putting them next to a step*, don't freak out or be surprised when Zoom takes a minute to work, make the whole world disabled.

I define cripping healing as any way a disabled person is defining the healing we want and need out of our expert knowledge in what works and doesn't work for us. We crip healing and health care when we stare back at the MIC and, instead of accepting what they offer us, demand and define what kinds of healing and health *we* want, on our own disabled terms.

There are a million ways this can manifest. Cripped healing might be about cure—but about a cripped cure, where disabled people are able to access pain meds, wound healing, cancer treatment, organ transplants, surgery, gender-affirming care, and the right to parent. These are things we are kept from being able to access every day, because the medical system doesn't believe we are "good candidates" or a doctor has never been taught how to help a post-polio,

---

* This was something Stacey Park Milbern did and wrote/spoke about (see Neil Genzlinger, "Stacey Milbern, a Warrior for Disability Justice, Dies at 33," *New York Times*, June 6, 2020, https://www.nytimes.com/2020/06/06/us/stacey-milbern-dead.html).

quad, bipolar, autistic, or Deaf person give birth. Or, because surgical and other treatments are taught to medical students on an assumed universal thin, abled, white body, no one knows how to take out our tumour or give us the chest we want.

Cripping healing can also be about divorcing *healing* from the idea of *fixing* disability. The MIC is obsessed with the idea of curing disabled body/minds, to the point where it's the only thing they can think to offer us, and if it's not possible, they shrug. But when I think about cripped healing in my own life, I think about my friends who threw away the braces doctors pushed on them as young physically disabled people with the promise that it would help them walk and instead chose to use wheelchairs as a much less painful, more pleasurable alternative. I think about the times I have crowdsourced treatment options from my sick and disabled queer community and gone to my specialist appointment armed with them, demanding and asking for the imaging and pain meds I wanted and asking them to document their denial in my chart when they denied it. I think about my choice to not follow up on the cortisol shots that will cause rebound pain and flares in my other joints after temporarily easing the pain in my own knee and instead choosing acupuncture, weed, ice packs, and the stretching method a fat femme friend on Instagram shared with me. I think about many things that have helped make my disabled life excellent—access tools, time, space, understanding, disabled and autistic community. My cane helps me walk and stand and get a seat and not fall over. Disabled community laughs with me and helps ease my pain days, knowledge shares, understands from the inside out what my life is like, never asks me to apologize for existing or to be grateful for crumbs. For many of us, cripping healing means, rather than a magic pill that will cure us as our big goal, we want adaptive devices, community, accessible work and housing, love, crip sexuality, sex ed and sex toys, shower chairs, personal care attendants, and many kinds of health care that offer more choices and options to live well in our disabled bodies, not correct them. And for many of us, cripping healing means we are seen as "bad," "demanding," "noncompliant" patients by the medical system. Depending on our other identities, privileges, and oppressions, the system can punish us for our noncompliance very harshly. Yet, as the autistic blog *Real Social Skills* put on a T-shirt beloved in autistic community, "Noncompliance Is a Social Skill."*

The work of cripping healing isn't easy. It's so hard to pull apart what actually sucks from what we've been taught to hate about our disabled body/minds. This is especially true when, like many disabled people, we have been isolated from other disabled people/ community to the point where we don't even know they exist, and/ or we have been taught to minimize or hide our disabilities, not ask for much, and be grateful for whatever we can get. But, as disabled Black lesbian feminist Audre Lorde wrote, "If I didn't define myself for myself, I would be crunched into other people's fantasies for me and eaten alive."[38]

What would a health care/healing system look like that loved and respected disabled people, where the first principle any healer was taught was that disability was both normal and awesome and that disabled people had full expertise and autonomy over our bodies?

What would medical schools look like if disabled, Mad, neurodivergent, and Deaf people wrote the textbooks, defined the diagnoses in the DSM, *threw out the* DSM?

When was the last time a health care provider asked you what your definition of healing or health was and how they could support you in it? Who asked what your goals were in meeting with them and how they could

---

* You can find the *Real Social Skills* blog at https://www.realsocialskills.org/ and if you want a shirt of your own, you can buy one here: https://www.bonfire.com/real-social-skills-t-shirt/.

respect your disabled body/mind? Who asked you to share your expertise on it?

Have you ever had a provider who did that?

Have you ever had a disabled, sick, Mad, neurodivergent, or Deaf health care provider?

If not, three guesses why that might be and the first two don't count.

THE FREE LIBRARY OF
BEAUTIFUL ADAPTIVE THINGS

I'm browsing through my email when my eye falls on an announcement from my local library, announcing that they are rolling out their new Library of Things. I am charmed and I read on. At the Library of Things* you can check out birding backpacks, fishing tackle and boxes, musical instruments, light therapy boxes (I live in Seattle, where we have no sun for six months of the year), and—wait for it—adaptive devices, or "Aids for Better Living for Individuals with Disabilities," as the website calls them.

I click the link and the website explains, in a big, accessible font and plain language, what everything is and what kinds of disabilities it might be useful for. "Dressing Stick: The long handle decreases the need for bending and it can be used for putting on all types of clothing. Ideal for anyone who has limited reach, arthritis or a broken hip" reads the description next to a cane-like device with a hook at the end that I certainly could use. There are all kinds of Things: adaptive controllers for Xboxes, playing cards with enlarged numbers, grabbers to help someone reach a dropped item without having

---

* In case you, too, want to check out this lovely program: https://www.trl.org/library-things, accessed April 30, 2021. Libraries of Things are a growing program—start one in your community!

to bend over, rose- and yellow-coloured glasses to help people with migraines and traumatic brain injuries (TBIs) use screens for longer, basic AAC (Augmentative and Alternative Communication) Devices for nonspeaking people, utensils with soft foam handles for people who have a hard time grasping, and utensils with weighted handles to steady hand tremors.

I'm blinking back tears. The Library is so beautiful. And I'm a forty-six-year-old disabled femme and this is the first time I've seen anything like it. It's so much easier to find information about right-to-die legislation pushing euthanasia for disabled people than an adaptive device library that might help make your life rock. There are many times I, and probably you, could have used The Library of Adaptive Things to Help My Disabled Life Be More Awesome—to try out a new device without paying for it, to use it for a little while if I only needed it temporarily, to not have to pay for it when I was poor, to be able to access it without having to have a series of arguments with my doctor or insurance provider that I should be able to access it.

It's so hard for many newly disabled or newly disabled-in-a-different-way people to try a wheelchair or some new meds or a jar opener—because of access to money and medicine, because of shame and internalized ableism that tells us that using any of those things is pathetic, but also because it's so hard to find information about adaptive technology at all. Have you ever tried to research using a new adaptive device? Was the info about it easy to find? Was it easy to find devices that were cute and affordable? Or were you hesitantly googling, getting overwhelmed, and putting down your computer, defeated?

And how often, if ever, have you had a doctor who was positive and encouraging and well informed and who offered you information about different adaptive tools, access hacks, or crip tricks? Mostly never, right? I have so many stories in my head of times when practitioners from community acupuncturists to rheumatologists reacted with shock, taken-abackness, and barely concealed disgust when they noticed my cane. They've said things like "How long have you been using ... THAT?" or "Well, we'll have to get rid of that ugly thing as soon as possible!" When I've subluxed my joints, it was other disabled people who offered that using forearm crutches or a wheelchair would give me mobility and take the weight off my knees, allowing them to heal—not doctors. I have a robust disabled community that can remind me that adaptive devices are super cool friends, but I still feel shitty after those encounters. I know it lands even more harshly on disabled people who don't have that kind of community, often delaying them from trying out a mobility device for months or years.

These encounters shape people's whole experiences of disability, turning what could be a neutral or joyful experience into an onerous burden. The Library creates a more playful, curious, and flexible space to explore disability and changing access needs, one where disability is a matter-of-fact everyday reality, so of course here is this publicly accessible free library of tools that can help you live it well.

CAN YOU WRITE ME A PRESCRIPTION FOR MY OWN ACCESSIBLE APARTMENT?

We're used to thinking of "healing" as specific treatments—surgery, pills, herbs, acupuncture. Those things are useful and important. But a cripped definition of healing would include *anything* that supports someone's disabled body/mind. My cane; my friend's garden bench chair they sit on while they weed; my heating pad and excellent ice packs; my friend's sensory friendly hijab[*]; the CRV my friend and his partner bought that can easily fit his wheelchair in the back; stim toys; my car with its disabled parking permit; the disabled

---

[*] http://rebirthgarments.com

parking spaces at the Grocery Outlet; the portable wheelchair at the protest; Zoom captions; the Autistic Black, brown, Indigenous, Asian and Mixed Race group I hang out in online; and my close and extended disabled BIPOC friend family who are available to bitch and vent and commiserate and troubleshoot and doula each other: none of these are healing in the "cure" sense. But all of these things do a lot to ensure my or someone else's chances of an excellent disabled life.

The items I use on that list are not things I knew I needed overnight. They emerged from a process of defining what healing looks for me as a disabled person, a process that's ongoing as I grow and my disabilities grow and change, too. It's a process whose goals are less about "curing my chronic illness"—which, like most of them, doesn't have a cure—and more about "less pain, adaptations that stretch my spoons, monitoring growths and illnesses early, and creating a sensory-friendly environment."

Figuring out those goals would not be possible without having disabled friends and disabled community who could do what disability justice activist Stacey Park Milbern referred to as "crip doulaing"[39]—the process by which disabled people mentor other disabled people in learning new disabled skills, from how to drive a wheelchair and negotiate with care attendants to how to have sex. She points out that until she invented the term in 2017, there was no word to describe this process of disabled-to-disabled mentorship and skill-sharing. And if you don't have words for something, it's hard to do it or imagine it's possible.

Both when we have a crip community and when we live in isolation, sick and disabled people are inventive and creative as we crip healing, and the ways we create to heal aren't ones that fit in most doctors' rule books. We know what we need, including when it looks wrong or silly or "crazy" to other people. The crip healing we create might be a freezer full of gluten-free frozen pizza and tater tots for high-pain, low-spoons days. It might be a Mad Map* or turning our phone off and going to the woods when we go into an altered state, temporal access[40], or a million hours of *The Office* cued up on Netflix. After fifteen months of severe back and hip pain, the sports medicine doctor I saw could only furrow her brow and push weight loss and more tests; I had a 90 percent pain reduction through a specific set of stretches† a disabled fat femme I knew mentioned on Instagram.

One of the biggest cornerstones of my own crip healing has been my ability to rent my own place—to live by myself, where I can cry as much as I need to, go make tea with no pants on, look weird, be tired, keep the place as clean as I need but also it's not a big deal if things get gross for a minute. Living alone has given me the autistic quiet I need to thrive, a place where I don't have to negotiate my access needs with anyone or mask. This is vital, for me and so many other Mad and neurodivergent folks. Yet you won't see the right to live alone in a messy, accessible, affordable apartment on any doctor's prescription pad.

CURE ≠ HEALING

In his book *Brilliant Imperfection: Grappling with Cure*, white disabled trans activist and writer Eli Clare writes about cure from every angle—how ideas of cure were invented by colonial Western doctors, settlers, and capitalists; what purposes cure serves and where it fails us; and what a disabled vision of a good life might be if we decentred cure. He writes, "At the center of cure lies eradication,"[41] of what he

---

* Mad Maps are documents similar to advance directives, written by Mad people describing what our altered states or crisis times look like and stating our needs, preferences, and boundaries for when we go into an altered state. See the Fireweed Collective or madqueer.org for more info and examples.

† In case you're wondering, it's the McKenzie Method. (See Robin McKenzie's series of books *Treat Your Own Back*, *Treat Your Own Hip*, etc.)

terms "brilliant imperfection"—all the skills, brilliance, ideas, art, community, and love that disabled people create because, not in spite, of our disabilities.

There are so many examples of the harm that comes from lifting up a cure model as the only way to fly, like how the MIC pushes treatments like ABA (applied behaviour analysis) on autistic children. ABA was first developed as a form of aversion therapy to "cure" queerness. It's now one of the most common treatments parents of newly diagnosed autistic kids are told they have to use on their kids. In ABA autistic kids are punished for exhibiting visibly autistic behaviour, like stimming, not making eye contact, or not speaking verbally. It literally uses the phrase "compliance training" in its pushing of autistic young people to stop acting autistic, setting us up for lifelong vulnerability to abuse—if you can't trust your gut when it wants you to act neurodivergent, how can you trust it when it tells you a partner or friend is abusing you? Although there are not a ton of studies backing this up—because the vast majority of funding for autism research is focused on "curing autism" rather than being led by or learning from neurodivergent people—there is a vast amount of anecdotal experiences shared among adult autistics reflecting on the lifelong damage ABA caused us and how we would have benefited much more from access to autistic community, access supports like alternative communication devices and sensory-friendly environments, love, and acceptance.*

Cure is also promised but just doesn't work! Telethons have been raising money to "cure" diseases for years but they're still here. And how many of us could trust the cures that are promised? Clare writes of his encounters with many doctors throughout his lifetime who promise that any day now, they'll be able to "cure" his cerebral palsy

---

* To learn more about this, check out the website *Stop ABA, Support Autistics: Advocating for Better Treatment of Autistic Individuals* (https://stopabasupportautistics.home.blog/).

and his retort to a recent one: "Not over my dead body. You can't even explain what happens between my brain and my muscles."[42] He writes of how telethons to "race for a cure" are so much more common and funded than events like Zoe's Race, an annual fundraiser held in Burlington, Vermont, where people roll, walk, and run, fundraising to make homes more disability accessible:

> Erika Nestor founded the event after she and her family renovated their home to make it more accessible for her disabled daughter, Zoe. Along the way, she learned just how expensive this kind of remodeling is and how little funding exists to help people make it happen ... Zoe's Race is motivated by the value of accessibility rather than cure. The money raised goes to something concrete, improving people's present-day lives, rather than something intangible centered on the future.[43]

Clare also complicates his anticure politics, writing about his friend with cancer who says, "I'm not at war with my body, but at the same time, I won't passively let my cancerous cells have their way with me."[44] He quotes disabled feminist thinker Susan Wendell, who says, writing about living with chronic pain, "Some unhealthy disabled people ... experience physical or psychological burdens that no amount of social justice can eliminate. Therefore, some very much want to have their bodies cured, not as a substitute for curing ableism, but in addition to it."[45]

AND YET: SOME OF US
NEED THE DAMN MEDS

Because that's the thing. We need both love and acceptance as we are as disabled *and* total access to the life-saving health care we need. Many of us really need access to western medicine—surgeries and transplants and drugs and chemo and wound care and equipment and western science. And some of us die without it.

On the night of April 19, 2021, I got a text message that my friend, Lucia Leandro "LL" Gimeno, had died. I finished this essay in the weeks after his death.*

It is hard to do justice to who LL was, but he touched literally thousands of people during his lifetime with his unapologetic, did-not-give-a-fuck/gave-many-fucks, loving, trans Afro-Latinx fat femme self. Both his giggle and his room-clearing laugh are some of the best laughs I have ever heard.

The child of a beautiful, fierce Latina lesbian mom who raised him and his twin in activist community in Jamaica Plain, Massachusetts, in the '80s, LL was always ready to do community safety patrols, hang out on the stoop, tear it up on the dance floor, sing along to Brandy, cook lavish meals, and listen to your problems on the phone. LL was present for so much foundational queer and trans BIPOC organizing—in the streets with groups like FIERCE, the Audre Lorde Project, and many others who created a new generation of queer/trans BIPOC organizing in the early 2000s when those organizing spaces were much less common than they are now. He moved to Seattle in 2016 to coordinate the Q/TPOC Birthwerq Project, organizing around queer and trans BIPOC reproductive justice issues like the right of Black trans women to parent. He was a bruj@, a theatre artist, and a honey healer.†

In 2017, soon after he moved to Seattle, LL got sick, ended up in the hospital, and discovered he was in late-stage kidney failure. He needed a kidney transplant, but for the next four years, doctors

---

* I am grateful to LL's mother, Antonieta Gimeno, and his twin, Yuisa Gimeno, for giving your blessing and support to me writing about LL, for loving him and fighting for him.

† For more about LL's work and legacy, check out https://www.facebook.com/QTPOCbirthwerq/, "The Reluctant Reproductive Justice Organizer and Birthworker" in *Radical Reproductive Justice: Foundations, Theory, Practice, Critique*, eds. Loretta J. Ross, Lynn Roberts, Erika Derkas, Whitney Peoples, and Pamela D. Bridgewater (New York: The Feminist Press, 2017), and https://www.ping chong.org/work/secret-survivors and https://www.facebook.com/lightonapathfollow/.

denied him one because according to them his BMI was "too high." This kind of fatphobic gatekeeping kills many fat people and is an issue fat activists have fought against for decades.

Despite all the bullshit, LL went to dialysis three times a week, held down multiple jobs, cooked, loved, made art, hung out with his friends, and did a huge amount of work organizing care, fighting for a transplant, and dealing with multiple hospital stays, doctors, and insurance.

I was a part of LL's care team and like all of us, I was devastated and shocked when he died. He had just taken new steps to get a kidney and was full of plans for writing, travelling, and healing. The day after he died, I sat in my rented birthday getaway crying and clutching my knees, wondering: *Could we have done more to help get him a kidney?* I was feeling guilty, going over all the times I hadn't been able to be there for him because I was on the road working or dealing with my own disability issues. My friend reminded me, "You all didn't fail. LL and everyone who loved him fought incredibly hard for him. The system failed. The system was the one who could get him a kidney."

It's often overt medical racism, ableism, fatphobia, and transphobic or sexist gatekeeping and abuse that steals our loved ones from us. But it can also be the more subtle kind of medical violence that kills, the death by a thousand cuts, the kind you can never sue for because it'll cost too much and besides, there's not one doctor or practitioner who failed—it's the whole system. LL kept getting infections and having to go to the hospital. He was in a lot of pain and so, so tired. A white doctor took herself off his care because when he asked her to speak to him respectfully, she said it made her feel "unsafe." Doctors put him on drugs and didn't explain the side effects or offer proactive care when he needed wound care. None of this was cripped healing. It was ableist, fatphobic, racist, and transphobic punishment.

The day he died, I was on the phone with many people who loved LL. We all said, they thought his fat, femme, Black Latinx trans life didn't matter. But we know how precious his life was, and we know how wrong they were. We all were so angry at the system that killed him, our beautiful Black Latinx trans disabled healer friend. We still are.

OUR WILD, PRECIOUS DISABLED LIVES: A MODEST PROPOSAL

In the days since LL passed, I've been thinking a lot about how many people the medical system has killed, how long people have been fighting against ableist medical abuse, and what needs to change so that nothing like this ever happens again.

And I'm going to be blunt: We need nothing less than a total remaking of the medical industrial complex into a health care and healing system where disabled bodies, minds, and lives are seen as valuable and perfect the way we are. We need a health care and healing system where we are known as experts on our own experience and people worthy of respect, autonomy, and care, not as pathologies. We need an end to the use of the BMI, and an end to the complete lack of even basic disability accessibility in health care settings, both of which shut people off from the health care access we need and deserve. We need an end to care rationing and triage where disabled, fat, BIPOC, trans, and older people are seen as less worthy of care.

Cripping healing can mean herbs and acupuncture and not going toward a cure as the only goal but asking and centring what we need and want in terms of access, disabled community, and support. However, it also must mean we get the western medical technologies that can literally save lives—surgery, vaccines, wound care, transplants, drugs, imaging—without gatekeeping. With COVID-19, we have seen the brilliant effects of mRNA vaccines deployed on a mass scale, for free—in First World countries who have access to them. We've also seen how common it's been for areas to think about or practise triaging, where disabled people are denied access to COVID care and vaccines. This has resulted both in massive disabled, fat, and elder activism* by groups like the NoBody Is Disposable Coalition and Disability Visibility Project fighting fiercely against medical rationing, and also in the deaths of disabled BIPOC people like Michael Hickson, a forty-six-year-old Black quadriplegic father of four who was denied care when he came down with COVID and died in Austin, Texas, in June 2020.[46]

As LL said, "It costs way less to provide free health care and education than it does to go elsewhere to bomb the shit out of some other country or lock people in prison."[47] We need an end to capitalist control of insurance and billing so that health care is no longer a luxury item you can only access if you can pay for it. We need a cripping of healing where not only are all forms of health care free, including adaptive equipment and accessible housing, work and play, but also funding and ableism aren't what fuels scientific research into treatments.

I've talked a lot of shit about the MIC's focus on magic pills in this essay, and I stand by that. What's also true is that there are few allopathic treatments for my autoimmune conditions (fibromyalgia, osteoarthritis, and atypical spondylitis) because they're seen by the medical system as conditions of little importance. Most of the people I know with chronic pain, autoimmune, and inflammatory conditions aren't white cis guys—we're some flavour of Black, brown, and broke people who have lived in brownfields, lead-filled cities, or rural communities with polluted groundwater, people who've

---

* For more info, check out Alice Wong's #HighRiskCA campaign and nobodyisdisposable.org.

survived a whole lot of rape, abuse, and violence. We're not rich, and drug companies will not make trillions of dollars creating some kind of miracle cure for our pain, so they focus on and fund skin whitening creams and impotence cures. Yet, like many, I would love The Science—all the science, including citizen science and science based in BIPOC communities' generations of traditional knowledge creation and research—to come up with pain meds that work, to research how trauma and environmental toxicity fuel the heightened pain response of my nervous system and to create something that would help it calm down. Cripping healing would mean both that disabled BIPOC would be able to be the scientists and healers using our disabled knowledge to do the research and try out the new treatments, and that we could use those treatments to feel less awful.

We need to cleanse medical schools and the MIC of the ableist, racist, transphobic, and fatphobic beliefs they teach and practise. From the beginning of medical training, students are taught to view disabled people as problems to be fixed. Things would be so different if disabled body/minds were not seen as pathologies but as unique bodies to be treasured, supported, and loved. Medical students aren't taught techniques to support disabled, BIPOC, queer and trans, and fat bodies. LL, like many fat people, was told that surgery and wound healing is "too difficult" in fat bodies for him to get a transplant. But I call bullshit. If fat, disabled, Black, and brown trans bodies were the norm, ways of doing surgery and aftercare on fat bodies would be practised and improved on the daily. If wheelchair users weren't seen as freaks, every dentist's chair and operating table would have to be built accessibly in order to be manufactured.

Cripping healing means believing our disabled lives are everyday and wonderful, worth saving and worth living. And it means changing every part of medical, health care, alternative healing, social security, housing and social and economic and cultural systems to reflect this. No more, and no less.

This may seem ambitious. But our disabled lives deserve everything. If in a pandemic year, people who always said access was "too hard" could move everything on Zoom, learn to caption and budget for ASL and build whole outdoor rooms, it's not much more of a stretch to demand that we turn the whole system that's killing us inside out.

Our lives are precious. And we deserve to be able to live them.

The System Isn't Broken, It's Working as Designed

Zena Sharman

MAPPING HEALTH SYSTEMS

If you had to draw a map of your experiences with the health system, what would it look like? Where would your map begin, and what landmarks would you include on it? Would you depict a straightforward path from one place to the next or a complex tangle of lines and broken or inaccessible pathways? Would you mark the dangerous or unknown places with fearsome monsters or mysterious mythical creatures? It might include paths to avoid at all costs, or treacherous paths that come with warning signs. Maybe your map would include shortcuts or hidden, more accessible pathways you created or learned about from others. My guess is each of our maps would look different, depending on who we are, where we live, and how we understand and relate to this system. For example, I live in Canada and have access to universal health care. Because my home is in a densely populated city I have greater access to acute and specialized hospital care than I would if I lived in a small rural or remote northern community. As a white cisgender nondisabled woman with financial privilege and a PhD, health care providers tend to treat me with respect, and I feel empowered to challenge them when they don't. When it comes to systems, context matters, as do our identities and social locations.

According to the World Health Organization, "A health system consists of all organizations, people and actions whose *primary intent* is to promote, restore or maintain health."[48] I like this definition because it's capacious enough to hold a whole range of things, like public or privately run hospitals and clinics, insurance companies, public health, health promotion, home and community care, complementary and alternative medicine, legislation, laws and policies, and caregiving provided by family and friends. My mental map of a health system also includes the places where people train to become health care providers, like medical or nursing schools. When I think of a health system, I tend to think big. My map feels like the kind that takes up a whole wall covered in paper and sticky notes, with strands of bright red yarn zigzagging across it in a web of interconnections. It gets even bigger when I zoom out to try and take in the whole medical industrial complex (MIC), an idea I explore in more detail later in this chapter.

When I was in graduate school, I studied how different health systems worked. This changed my experiences as a patient because it helped me understand why something that happened in an individual interaction—say, a short, rushed visit with my doctor—was shaped by the history and inner workings of a much larger system. In Canada, most doctors work as independent contractors who bill the public health care system for their services. Some of them (just under half, as of 2017) get paid through a piecework model called "fee-for-service" medicine.[49] Doctors working under this model bill the government for individual interactions with patients, like an immunization or an assessment for a specific illness or disease. It's a way of getting paid that's been criticized for incentivizing seeing more patients in less time instead of rewarding doctors for the quality of their care or their relationships with patients as whole, complex people.[50]

Fee-for-service medicine is, in turn, a model entangled with the history of universal health care in Canada as it came out of a compromise between government and doctors. Universal health care in Canada was initially met with fierce opposition from powerful groups like the Canadian Medical Association and the American Medical Association, who were afraid it would spark similar changes in the United States.[51] They used Red Scare–inflected rhetoric like "socialism" and "communism" in their ultimately unsuccessful fight against a government program they saw as limiting doctors' independence and entrepreneurialism.

In Saskatchewan, the Canadian province where universal health care was first introduced, doctors backed by powerful interest groups protested by going on strike for three weeks in 1962. When tracing these histories, it's important to remember there also was a smaller group of doctors who worked in collaboration with activists, socialists, trade unionists, and agrarian radicals to organize community clinics and counterprotests during the strike.[52] The strike ended when the provincial government and striking doctors arrived at an agreement that included fee-for-service medicine; this form of payment preserved doctors' ability to remain as self-employed professionals in the publicly funded health system.[53] While some doctors today are paid through alternative models like salaries or capitation (a monthly payment based on the number of patients in their practice), fee-for-service medicine remains a dominant way of paying doctors in Canada.

The fee-for-service model is one of many reasons my doctor might have rushed through our too-short appointment. Maybe he was running behind because his previous appointment went long and it had been hours since he last took a break, or the time it takes to use the clinic's electronic medical record cut into the already-limited time he has for face-to-face visits with patients. Perhaps his medical training taught him to prioritize efficiency and diagnosis over listening and connection. He may have spent less time with me because he was inclined to dismiss my concerns, a reflection of the ways health care providers sometimes gaslight patients. My goal here is to put our interaction in the context of a larger health system with its own history and logics, not find a single cause for why my doctor was in such a hurry. There are rarely single causes when you're dealing with something as complex as a health system.

To speak of a health system is to speak in abstractions and multiplicities while at the same time describing something vast and concrete. There is no single health system; there are many of them made up of multiple components, each shaped by the history and context of its location. These systems don't work seamlessly. They have fractures, breaks, gaps, and internal contradictions and conflicts that leave people with inadequate care or no care at all.

In Canada, for example, where universal health care first developed within a hospital-centred paradigm, there's inadequate and inequitable access to mental health care and a lack of public coverage for things like most dental and vision care and out-of-hospital prescription drugs.[54] The Canadian health system also excludes whole groups of people, like those with precarious or no status (e.g., people who have overstayed visas or whose refugee claims have been rejected, most temporary foreign workers) and provides inadequate coverage to people who have made refugee claims or who are incarcerated in detention centres.[55]

In the United States, access to health insurance is often tied to employment, marriage, and citizenship. While the Affordable Care Act has improved many people's ability to access health care, many others remain underinsured or uninsured and can't afford the health care they need. Research has shown this disproportionately affects trans people, especially those who are Indigenous, Black, and/or Latinx, living in the South, or without citizenship status.[56] How health systems are designed has implications for who has access to care and who gets left out. These gaps are rarely accidental.

Every person reading this book is in a place with its own health system (or systems). You're in relationship with this system and are intimately acquainted with where it works and where it harms or fails to care for you. I'm writing these words in Vancouver, Canada. When I picture the health system as I experience it I think of the community health centre near my apartment where I've been a patient for almost twenty years and where I can see my family doctor or a nurse practitioner. I picture the hospital where my kid was born with the help of a midwife. I think of the dentist's office I can afford to visit regularly because my day job offers supplemental private insurance that covers the cost of dental care. I picture the faces of all the therapists I've paid for privately because it was the only way I could access mental health care that felt supportive to me as a queer person. I imagine the many home care workers who cared for my mother when she was sick and dying, highly skilled and chronically underpaid work that kept my mom out of the long-term care facility she desperately wanted to avoid.

These are all nodes in a much larger health system I've been embedded in all my life, whether or not I was conscious of it. Health systems have a way of fading into the background that can give them a taken-for-granted quality. This isn't because we always trust the system will be there for us when we need it; rather, it's because many of us have internalized the idea that the way the health system operates is somehow normal or natural. It's just the way things are.

Many people live, suffer, and sometimes die inside the harm and violence of "it's just the way things are." This taken-for-grantedness can also limit our ability to imagine what kinds of change might be necessary or desirable to create a health system capable of meeting LGBTQ+ people's needs. To change a system, we need to be able to perceive it.

THE MEDICAL INDUSTRIAL COMPLEX

Health systems are built around a set of assumptions about health and illness, disability, and cure, who is and isn't deserving of care, and who does and does not have a "good" body. Though it's often held up as a universal good and something to strive for, health is not a neutral, objective, or universal concept. The meaning of "health" is constructed and shifts depending on where and when it's created, and by whom. Notions of cure aren't neutral, either. Disabled genderqueer writer and activist Eli Clare describes cure as "a widespread ideology centred on eradication," one that "operates in relationship to violence" and is grounded in ableist assumptions about what's normal and natural.[57] Further, the designation of some people, communities, and populations as "healthy" and others as "unhealthy" is entangled with systemic oppression and social control.

For example, despite scientific evidence to the contrary, fatter bodies are frequently associated with risk and ill health, leading to weight stigma and weight bias that undermine fat people's ability to access quality health care.[58] Disabled bodies are often perceived as tragic, broken, or in need of cure because of the ableism that permeates so much of the health system. As disability ethicist Heidi L. Janz points out, ableism "often presents as 'common sense'" in medicine.[59] The sexualities of gay, bisexual, queer, and other men who have sex with men are framed as risky behaviours to be surveilled, controlled, or managed, with little consideration of pleasure or the structural and material conditions of people's lives.[60] Assumptions like these shape the design of our health systems and the content of health care provider education and training. They limit the possibilities available to queer and trans people for health and healing inside a system that wasn't created with us in mind.

My mental map of the health system grew even bigger when I was introduced to the concept of the medical industrial complex (MIC), as interpreted by activists, organizers, and healers whose analyses are grounded in healing justice and disability justice. I need to zoom out wider to perceive this map in its entirety because the MIC encompasses and shapes the health system yet is broader than it alone. As a concept, the vastness of the MIC is both incredibly useful and potentially overwhelming. It's useful because it helps me understand the workings of the health system and identify potential sites of change in that system. It also sometimes leaves me feeling like the stereotypical conspiracy theorist, arms waving frantically in front of my wall-sized map while I shout, "It's all connected!" And it is, because that's how systems work.

Some of you might be familiar with variations on the idea of an industrial complex—the military-industrial complex, for example, or the prison industrial complex. What they have in common is the idea of an interconnected set of relationships among different entities (e.g., groups, companies, entire industries), underpinned by shared beliefs, motives, and a drive for profit, power, and social control. The concept of the MIC was first introduced in a 1969 article published in the monthly bulletin of an activist group called the Health Policy Advisory Center or Health/PAC; Barbara and John Ehrenreich later elaborated on the idea in a 1970 book called *The American Health Empire: Power, Profits and Politics*.[61] These activists critiqued a profit-driven health system in which health was seen as both a commodity and an economic good.

Today, the MIC is a vast, interconnected system encompassing a range of institutions, professions, sites, and sectors. The conceptualization of the MIC I explore here is grounded in the work of queer, trans, disabled, and Black, Indigenous, and people of colour activists, organizers, and healers at the vanguard of movements for healing and disability justice. Their analysis of the MIC is broader than the original in that it focuses on how the MIC functions as a system of social control through its connections to colonialism, racism, ableism, and other forms of oppression.

Healing justice organizers and practitioners Anjali Taneja, Cara Page, and Susan Raffo, whose collaborative work seeks to document and disrupt the MIC, articulate these connections:

> from the beginnings of the institution of colonization and slavery, the state has systematically determined who is "normal," "healthy," "diseased," and "dangerous" as a way of determining access to its rights and benefits. The medical industrial complex emerged as an extension of policing and state violence to control the biology and healing practices and to define the line between "normal" and not.[62]

Writer and educator Mia Mingus offers a visual map of the MIC that illustrates these ideas at a system level.[63] Her map includes health care (hospitals, clinics, health centres, etc.); medical schools; pharmaceutical companies; the mental health industry; drug addiction facilities and programs; non-western and alternative healing; the alternative and natural medicines industry; assisted living; disability services and programs; assistive devices, equipment, and services; nonprofits; insurance companies; and the prison industrial complex.

Tying all this together are MIC's core motivations: eugenics, charity and ableism, population control, and desirability. By mapping the MIC in this way, Mingus is "calling attention to the systematic targeting of oppressed communities under the guise of care, health and safety."[64] She is careful to point out that many people access life-saving or life-sustaining care, treatment, and technologies inside the MIC. She explains her intention in mapping the MIC is to name it as a system, so as to enable transformation of this system and the building of alternatives to it.

The health system often invisibilizes LGBTQ+ people, stigmatizes us, or fails to meet our needs; this can result in harm and unmet need. We're sometimes left feeling like we have to contort ourselves to fit a system not designed for us, whether it's by scratching out the limiting categories on an intake form and adding our own or sharing system navigation strategies like which emergency room to go to if you're in crisis—or ways to avoid the emergency room altogether. We're adept at getting what we need in the face of enormous systemic barriers, yet we can still be left feeling like outliers: wrong, deviant, broken.

This is no accident; it's a property of the system. Mordecai Cohen Ettinger, the disabled queer/genderqueer founding director of activist group Health Justice Commons, emphasizes, "Much of the MIC's control is derived from the production and amplification of social division—that which is 'normal' and 'valuable' vs. that which is 'deviant, sick, ill, or disposable.'"[65] He notes that this both generates and amplifies systemic oppression, especially racialized and gendered ableism, and leads to high degrees of medical surveillance and control of those deemed "deviant" by the MIC.

In a talk on disrupting the MIC, Taneja and Page outline its core assumptions, functions, and impacts.[66] The ideal "healthy" body in the MIC is wealthy, white, cisgender, heterosexual, nondisabled, and male. Proximity to this ideal shapes beliefs about who is most deserving of access to quality, dignified care, as well as whether or not people and communities can access this kind of care. Institutions within the MIC function to extend state control and violence in how they surveil, police, and erase bodies that don't fit this narrow ideal. Bodies outside this ideal—including queer and trans bodies—are more likely to be criminalized, pathologized, and deemed ugly, undesirable, expendable, or unfit to survive. The MIC emphasizes cure, as delivered through western or allopathic medicine in a context of disease-based capitalism, while simultaneously limiting, disdaining, or criminalizing practitioners outside these models of care.

The historical and present-day workings of the MIC are too vast to discuss in detail here, as are the forms of medical violence they inflict on people, groups, and communities. Instead, I offer several examples to illustrate what the MIC looks like in action, in the hope that they will inspire you to notice how the MIC shows up in your life. This practice of naming and noticing can be helpful in our efforts to make sense of and transform the health system; it can also be protective against messages you might receive inside the system that tell you that you're broken or not credible, or that it's all your fault.

The Flexner report: How a report from 1910 is still shaping medicine today (and why I'm mad about it)

In university and college settings, the phrase "first-generation" is often used to refer to the experiences of people who are the first in their family to access postsecondary education. Medical students taught me a different meaning of this term, one that took some of them (and also me!) by surprise: to some people, being a "first-generation" medical student means being the first person in your family to go to medical school. Implicit in this is the reality that, according to some studies, somewhere around 15 to 20 percent of medical students have parents or other relatives who are doctors.[67] Many more come from affluent families. In the United States, around three-quarters of medical students come from higher-income families, a distribution that hasn't changed in thirty years.[68] In 2020, 7.7 percent of US medical students reported annual family incomes of $500,000 or more; the median family income of US medical students was $130,000 a year, more than double the median income of US families.[69] The picture is similar in Canada, where studies have shown that the majority of medical school applicants and medical students come from higher-income families.[70]

Medical schools have been described as "racialized organizations" where "current organizational structures and processes often serve to entrench, not dismantle, racial inequities."[71] In the United States, Indigenous, Black, and Latinx people are underrepresented among medical students, and white men make up the majority of medical school faculty and active physicians.[72] These trends are similar in Canada, where Indigenous and Black people are underrepresented among medical students, as are students from rural areas or lower-income families.[73] Disabled people are also underrepresented in medicine and experience ableism in their educational environments.[74] As queer community-based physician and organizer Nanky Rai writes, a medical school admissions process that "works to uphold colonialism and intersecting class, race, gender and other forms of power in society sets up a vicious cycle of medical violence."[75]

When I look at these statistics, I notice patterns of privilege underlying who has access to medical education. While becoming a doctor is far from the only way to provide health care for your community, medicine is a useful case study for understanding why there often seems to be big gaps between who gets to become a doctor and which groups and communities experience the most significant health disparities. If you've never had a doctor who looks like you, it's no accident. It's a by-product of fundamentally inequitable pathways into medical education situated within the larger dynamics of the MIC.

The answer to the question of why so many groups are underrepresented in medicine is complex and multifaceted, but we can find one part of it in a report that's over a hundred years old yet is still shaping medical education today. In 1910, an educational reformist named Abraham Flexner published a report called *Medical Education in the United States and Canada* (more commonly known as the Flexner report) that evaluated more than 150 medical schools in the United States and Canada. At the time, medical education looked a lot different than it does today: there were "no standards across schools for admission, curriculum, or graduation." [76] While today we might associate medical schools with universities, in Flexner's day they took many forms, including as privately run commercial enterprises.

Although modern medical science was gaining prominence, if you went to medical school in the early 1900s, you might also study subjects like osteopathy, chiropractic medicine, homeopathy, or botanical and herbal medicine. In addition to many schools serving white men, there were seven medical schools located at historically Black colleges and universities (HBCUs) and a number of women's medical colleges.

Flexner's review of medical schools was commissioned by the Carnegie Foundation. The Carnegie Foundation was funded by Andrew Carnegie, one of the richest men in America. His fortunes came from investments in industries like oil, iron, and steel, a legacy that includes the deaths of workers at the hands of violent strike-breakers.[77] In 1900, Carnegie made $480 million from the sale of the Carnegie Steel Company.[78] He then shifted his focus to philanthropy. Around this time, Carnegie and other multimillionaires like John D. Rockefeller and Russell Sage "created new [philanthropic] institutions that would exist in perpetuity and support charitable giving in order to shield their earnings from taxation."[79] The creation of this system of philanthropic foundations is deeply tied up with the emergence of the modern nonprofit sector and a charity model rooted in hierarchy, "deservingness," and attempts at social control disguised as betterment, all of which have everything to do with how the MIC operates.

The Carnegie Foundation's interest in medical education was prompted by a request from the American Medical Association (AMA)'s Council on Medical Education, who had conducted their own survey of US medical schools in 1906. The AMA had "proclaimed as semiofficial policy the goal of eliminating commercial [medical] schools and reducing the number of new physicians produced each year."[80] The AMA also had long-standing racist and sexist policies that served to exclude Black physicians and women physicians from participation in medical societies.[81] In response, Black physicians founded their own organization, the National Medical Association, in 1895.[82] During the same era, the AMA "worked state by state to outlaw abortion to drive midwives from medical care and to establish regular doctors as the sole source of medical care."[83] This was a deliberate effort to eliminate competition from midwives, who had traditionally assisted pregnant people with birth and abortions.

In an article on the racialized, gendered, and regional implications of the Flexner report, scholar Moya Bailey notes that Flexner thought the United States needed "fewer and better doctors" who his report represents as "white men of means, privilege, and Northern sensibilities."[84] In practice, this looked like proposing to close all the women's medical colleges and most medical colleges at HBCUs where Black doctors were being trained. Flexner also called into question the then-common practice of arranging medical school academic calendars around seeding and harvest time, which excluded students from rural communities.

Flexner's efforts at reform were rooted in a desire to streamline, standardize, and modernize medical education. He emphasized scientific medicine and argued that "every medical school should be integrated into a university with a sufficient endowment and a university hospital."[85] To offset the costs of this expensive educational model, Flexner "encouraged philanthropy from wealthy individuals and foundations as a key source of revenue for medical schools and universities."[86] This increased medical education's dependence on philanthropy and created barriers for medical schools not connected with or desirable to wealthy white donors. For example, in 1919 Flexner persuaded the Rockefeller Foundation to donate $50 million to implement his report's recommendations, which "brought about the transformation of many medical schools" in line with his vision.[87] Flexner's financial and infrastructural requirements created "impossible benchmarks" for medical schools at HBCUs, who were expected to demonstrate "the same level of institutional resources that were expected of predominantly white medical schools."[88]

At a time when many medical students were admitted with a high school education or less, Flexner advocated for prospective students to have at least two years of college and knowledge of chemistry, biology, and physics. As Bailey points out, "These core subjects, with the addition of mathematics and writing, remain the core requirements for medical school admission to this day."[89] These requirements functionally excluded students who couldn't afford or access the requisite college education and contributed to income disparities in access to medical education reminiscent of the contemporary ones I cited earlier.

The Flexner report contributed to the closure of many medical schools. In the early 1900s, there were over 160 medical schools; by 1928, there were only seventy-six.[90] Schools that educated Black people, women, working-class people, and those located in medically underserved regions like the US South or Atlantic Canada were particularly impacted by these closures. Buttressed by his emphasis on modern scientific medicine, Flexner also "advocated for the closing of nearly eighty percent of all the contemporary [medical education] programs in homeopathy, naturopathy, eclectic therapy, physical therapy, osteopathy, and chiropractic."[91]

The Flexner report contributed to the closure of five out of the seven medical schools located at HBCUs. Ultimately, only two medical schools at HBCUs—Howard and Meharry—remained open. In a recent study examining the impacts of these closures on the number of Black medical graduates in the United States, Kendall M. Campbell and colleagues found the five closed medical schools at HBCUs "might have collectively provided training to an additional 35,315 graduates by 2019," potentially resulting in a 29 percent increase in the number of graduating Black physicians in the United States in 2019 alone.[92]

The Flexner report also affected women's ability to access medical training. Shari L. Barkin and colleagues point out that in the period just before the Flexner report, women physicians had a "significant presence in many parts of the United States."[93] Women created and led their own medical schools and hospitals after all-male medical institutions refused to admit them—in 1900, the United States had seven women's medical colleges. By 1930, only one (the Woman's Medical College of Pennsylvania) remained. The overall number of women graduating from medical school in the United States declined to an all-time low (2.9 percent) by 1915; women made up less than 5 percent of medical graduates until the 1970s.

These gender dynamics look different today—since 2003, similar proportions of women and men have applied to, entered, and graduated from US medical schools, and over 50 percent of US medical students were women in 2019.[94] In Canada, over half of doctors under the age of forty are women and it's projected the physician pool will be equally split among women and men by 2030. However, medical students and physicians still face gender discrimination, sexual harassment, and sexual violence at school and work.[95] Trans, nonbinary, and gender-diverse medical students are confronted with the harms and challenges of navigating a cisnormative medical culture.[96]

Although it was written over 100 years ago, the impacts of the Flexner report continue reverberating through medicine. As Bailey astutely observes, "The latent white supremacy embedded within Flexner's report continues to colour medicine more than 100 years later."[97] When trying to make sense of disparities in access to medical education and why your doctors might rarely share your identities and lived experiences, it's important to consider the history that brought us to where we are today.

Pandemics, public health, and policing

Another way to understand how the historical origins and assumptions built into a system shape its present-day functioning is by looking at the institution of public health. The Canadian Public Health Association defines public health as "the organized effort of society to keep people healthy and prevent injury, illness and premature death" through a combination of programs, services, and policies.[98] This book was written during the COVID-19 pandemic, a time when public health played a prominent and highly visible role in managing and responding to the pandemic, often in concert with the police and the legal system. I'm writing these words in April 2021 just days after the Minister of Public Safety and Solicitor General in my home province issued an emergency order empowering the Royal Canadian Mounted Police (RCMP) to set up police checkpoints on highways to deter "nonessential" travel. This decision will disproportionately affect racialized communities who consistently experience the harms of overpolicing. History matters here: the RCMP originated in the late nineteenth century to violently enforce Canada's racist, colonial policies against Indigenous peoples. They continue upholding genocidal policies today, such as the removal of Indigenous land and water defenders from their sovereign territory, yet as recently as June 2020 the RCMP's national leader publicly denied the existence of systemic racism in their organization.

In many Canadian provinces and cities, governments declared lockdowns, granting police "sweeping powers to enforce public health measures and local by-laws that instituted fines, checkpoints, border closures, curfews, entire lockdowns of cities and towns, and ID checks."[99] COVID noncompliance "snitch lines" also emerged across the country in the early months of the pandemic, with over thirty in place by June 2020. The Canadian Civil Liberties Association estimates that between April and June 2020, over 10,000 tickets were issued or charges laid related to COVID-19, resulting in over $13 million in fines in Canada during this three-month period alone.[100] These fines spiked during the second wave of the pandemic. For example, in British Columbia, 1,584 fines were handed out between August 2020 and March 2021, a significant increase over the approximately twenty-two fines issued during the first several months of the pandemic. Quebec has been one of the most punitive provinces in Canada, "issuing over 16,000 COVID-19 tickets, totalling more than $24 million in fines."[101] Scholar-activists Alexander McClelland and Alex Luscombe point to this mobilization of policing agents as an example of "further 'policification'—that is, the expansion of police power into non-traditional roles that are better covered by other kinds of institutional actors."[102]

These forms of surveillance, criminalization, and punishment disproportionately affect Black, Indigenous, and other racialized communities, as well as migrants, LGBTQ+ people, disabled people, youth, people who are confined to institutions such as prisons, and people who are precariously housed or involved in informal economies like sex work or the drug trade. As Black feminist activists Robyn Maynard and Andrea J. Ritchie observe, "pandemic policing extends and expands pre-existing policing patterns" that criminalize and harm these communities.[103] Speaking directly to the impact on Black communities, they point to the fact that "Blackness itself has historically been framed as a threat, both to public health and broader society."[104] To believe this would shift during a public health crisis of this magnitude is, as Maynard and Ritchie put it, "magical thinking."

The authors of the *We Can't Police Our Way Out of the Pandemic: Lessons for Abolition* report frame public health both "as a social institution and a practice," one that constructs the public as "groups that are not deemed to pose a threat of infection."[105] Here we see the logics of the MIC at work, where some groups are excluded from "the public" by the risk they are assumed to pose to those who fit easily within the definition of public. As queer scholar-activist Gary Kinsman reminds us, "We must always ask who is the 'public,' and whose health is being protected?"[106]

Here it's helpful to look to the historical origins of the institution and practice of public health. Colonizers who came to North America from Europe brought with them lessons they'd learned from the bubonic plague in the fourteenth century. For centuries, they relied on quarantine and isolation to manage epidemics of diseases like smallpox, yellow fever, cholera, and typhus. These deadly viruses and bacteria had devastating effects on Indigenous communities who lacked immunity to them and whose ability to withstand these illnesses was hampered by the health impacts of colonial violence like warfare, starvation, and forced removal from their lands.[107] By the nineteenth century, public health officials were utilizing familiar-sounding tactics like mandatory isolation and confinement of infected people, compulsory vaccination, fines, mandatory reporting of infected patients by doctors, contact tracing, and other forms of surveillance.[108]

These tactics relied on a narrow, exclusionary definition of the "public," leading to the stigmatization, targeting, incarceration, or forcible inoculation of groups thought to be at higher risk of disease, like Indigenous people, Black people, racialized migrants, poor people, sex workers, and LGBTQ+ people. In Canada, for example, an entire network of segregated "Indian Hospitals" was established as part of colonial, assimilationist efforts to control tuberculosis transmission among Indigenous peoples. [109] And while "Typhoid Mary's" nickname might be well-known by some, I suspect fewer people know she was a working-class woman named Mary Mallon who spent the last twenty-three years of her life forcibly confined to a quarantine facility on an island near the Bronx.[110]

The definition of the "public" that structures the institution of public health is entangled with histories of systemic oppression and the targeting and stigmatization of specific groups. We can observe this dynamic at work over centuries, including more recently during the AIDS crisis and in the criminalization of people with HIV. In Canada, for example, over 200 people have been criminally prosecuted for alleged HIV nondisclosure since 1989, with intensified impacts on Black, Indigenous, and people of colour; women; and people without citizenship. As with other forms of criminalization, this can have devastating effects on people's lives.[111] These same dynamics are at work today during the COVID-19 pandemic and affirm the necessity of interrogating the carceral logics shaping the institution and practice of public health, as well as how these same dynamics show up in medicine and the MIC.

"EVERY SYSTEM IS PERFECTLY DESIGNED TO GET THE RESULTS IT GETS"

For a long time, I thought of health care as a broken system that needed fixing. I believed we could fix the system by making health care more inclusive of and affirming to LGBTQ+ people. This would make it easier for our community to access health care and contribute to our overall health and well-being. There is a truthfulness to this perspective—the current system can be so fundamentally unwelcoming and harmful to queer and trans people that efforts to make it more inclusive and affirming might reduce harm. When done well, as some providers, groups, and organizations already are, providing inclusive and affirming LGBTQ+ health care can be life sustaining, healing, and transformational for the people receiving care.

Where my perspective has shifted—where I've realized my own thinking fell short—is in how I comprehend the health system *as a system*, with its own history, logics, and inbuilt assumptions. The idea that the system is broken presumes the existence of a prior state of wholeness and functioning that needs to be restored—if we can just get back to this place, things will get better. Learning from the transformative justice (TJ) movement helped shift my understanding of this dynamic, in how, instead of having as a goal trying to return things to the way they were before the harm was caused (something foundational to some restorative justice programs), TJ believes that in order to build safer communities we have to transform the conditions that lead to violence in the first place—what conditions lead someone to steal, rape, or otherwise cause harm, like poverty or sexism.[112]

As I've engaged more deeply in learning about transformative justice, abolition, healing justice, disability justice, and related concepts like the MIC, I've come to understand the insufficiency of the idea that our goal should be to fix a broken health system. It's insufficient because it bypasses the truth that the system isn't broken; it's working as designed. It was never built for LGBTQ+ people, and has often been complicit in, or the driver of, efforts to discipline, control, or eradicate our unruly and deviant bodies. As they say in the health care quality field, "Every system is perfectly designed to get the results it gets."[113]

LGBTQ+ people consistently report experiencing discrimination in health care settings and face persistent barriers to accessing health care. Some people avoid health care altogether because the risk of being harmed by homophobia, biphobia, transmisogyny, transphobia, racism, ableism, fatphobia, and other forms of discrimination feels greater than the health concern that might drive them to seek care in the first place. All of this contributes to the health disparities faced by the LGBTQ+ community, disparities that are worse for anyone whose body bears the brunt of systemic oppression. This is no accident; it is a predictable outcome of a health system rooted in normative ideals of health and illness that often exclude and harm those who fail to conform to those ideals.

I have come to understand more fully and urgently than I used to that our health system needs to be fundamentally transformed to provide the liberatory care I dream of for LGBTQ+ people. That's why I'm inviting you to think with me about the health system: to practise perceiving it as a system, interrogate its history and underlying assumptions and their implications for LGBTQ+ health, and begin imagining ways to transform or work outside of the existing system in order to enable our collective survival, flourishing, and liberation.

Queer and trans people have a long-standing practice of sharing tips and strategies for navigating the health system and figuring out how to survive when confronted with gaps we might otherwise fall into. I'm reminded of T Fleischmann's story of searching for answers to a persistent health issue doctors couldn't figure out and finding the answer at a house party/community bail bond fundraiser. There, a trans woman with experience taking similar hormones explained to them that it was a side effect of Spironolactone. About this encounter, Fleischmann writes,

> "Who told you?" I ask. "How did you figure this out?" And it's always friends of friends, where knowledge like this originates, accumulating like the residual of the pills, one at a time, until eventually something clicks together in the social and it can be known.[114]

That "click" of knowing and sharing what we know is one of the queer and trans community's superpowers and core survival strategies. In this spirit, I'm curious what it might look like if we actually created and shared our own maps of the health systems we interact with, on our own or together with our communities, including all the shortcuts, side paths, and secret tunnels we use to make our way through those systems. So many trans, fat, Black and Brown, and sick and disabled people already are doing this kind of mapping—from informal networks where disabled people "crip doula" and share skills, knowledge about treatments, and strategies for navigating (or bypassing) the health system, to fat community–created lists of fat-friendly providers, to the trans community networks like the ones Fleischmann writes of above.

What could we learn by better understanding the historical roots and ideas built into the health system? How might we situate our maps in relation to the MIC and practise naming the implicit assumptions that often render the system so dangerous in the first place? LGBTQ+ people are already adept at navigating through and around the health system. My hope is that reading this chapter will offer you useful and perhaps new ways of thinking about this system as you traverse or deliberately work outside of it.

As we dream into the kinds of care we hope to create for ourselves and our communities, I'm also curious how our maps of the system might change—maps are subjective, after all, and reflect the perspectives of their creators. What routes to health and healing do you want to create for yourself and your community? How do you want to feel during the journey? How might we work together to transform the difficult or scary places on your maps into somewhere safer, more beautiful, and that you genuinely want to move toward? How are we already doing this work, and what do we need to make it even bigger and more beautiful?

the seven sacred ways of healing

jaye simpson

/let it out/

releasing only
as much as i thought
they could hold;
kept asking "why
did you do that to me"
thru clamped jaw
& gritted teeth—

/don't ask why/

/let it out/
/let it out/

tear through
rawing throat,
saliva & blood
bubbling
wild prairie fire
cacophony.

/there will never be an answer/

                                                          /let it out/
                                                          /let it out/
                                                          /let it out/

her hand presses
deep into my breast,
pinpointed compression
my chest billows
                    /tell them what they did/

                                                          /let it out/
                                                          /let it out/
                                                          /let it out/
                                                          /let it out/

head thrown back
screams ripping out of my throat
faster than i can breathe,
eyes strained—
hemorrhage spread
across my sclera.
                    /you will never get to ask why/

                                                          /let it out/
                                                          /let it out/
                                                          /let it out/
                                                          /let it out/
                                                          /let it out/

i cough blood &
retch, i am told
i am letting go.
                    /tell them what they did/

                                                        /let it out/
                                                        /let it out/
                                                        /let it out/
                                                        /let it out/
                                                        /let it out/
                                                        /let it out/

i can no longer lift
my arms, Zhigaag takes
my place punching the bag,
our screams synchronizing,
letting go breaks everything.
                            /this will follow them/

                                                        /let it out/
                                                        /let it out/
                                                        /let it out/
                                                        /let it out/
                                                        /let it out/
                                                        /let it out/
                                                        /let it out/
                                                        /let it out/

final screams
dying with vocal fry
& tears tinged red,
ribbon skirt pooling
around my crumpled form
hands clawing at chest
Zhigaag's screams billow out now.
                        /they will know what it meant/

When I was approached with an opportunity to return to my traditional homelands for the first time in my life, I was terrified. What if the community I am from rejects me in my womanhood, therefore erasing my claim to Indigeneity? I would lose this important pillar of who I am and would have to forfeit my historical and Ancestral responsibilities. I had already lost kinship with my Maternal Grandmother because of her transphobic rhetoric, but she is no traditionalist.

The need to be claimed outweighed the fear of loss, even though I had told myself I was okay with not returning to my home territories for a while. I couldn't handle grieving my relationship with the land my family had kinship with anymore. It didn't seem fair for me to mourn my displacement if I wasn't taking this opportunity to return.

So, I returned. I learned much more than I ever anticipated, especially the generosity of my peoples and the land. I also learned of my own classism and how my fear was based on my access to academic social justice language and rhetoric. My own cousins, who had no knowledge of politically correct and affirming language, had a practice of care, kinship, and community so developed and inviting it was beyond anything I had seen in Vancouver's own Queer Community. I saw Indigenous trans women employed at the Band Office. I saw Indigenous trans women leading Women's Water Ceremonies. I saw Indigenous trans women valued so deeply, something I was told I would never find here.

I was there for a Women's Healing Camp and it was here that I came face to face with my own peoples' practice of healing: no one can heal alone; when one is hurting, we all are. In a tent in the Manitoba June heat, a dozen other women and I screamed in unison, rocking back and forth on mats, kicking and screaming, throwing up bile in our collective screaming.

It was the most radical and affirming healing I had ever participated in. The years of therapy and counsellors, years of white women telling me I am resilient, were nothing compared to having my cousins hold me as I screamed.

I had begun asking why, why did I experience this pain? Why did I have to be subjected to so much horrific violence at such a young age? An Aunty guiding me through the Ceremony took my face in her hands and told me I would never get to ask why; I would only ever be able to tell folks what had happened.

This was a revolutionary realization: no matter what, I would never know justification for my abuse, but that didn't mean I had to keep it to myself. For the first time in my life, I was allowed to scream until my throat was raw, loudly mourning the parts of my life that were torn from me.

Through this Ceremony, I experienced a terrifying truth: we had lost the ability to collectively grieve with our kin; instead, we are conditioned to silently cope with the trauma on our own, taught that our burdens were ours alone.

To spend time being held by my own family, folks I was kept from for years due to foster care and forced assimilation, and for us to collectively scream, affirmed my instinctual need to cry out in times of trauma. For years I was told I couldn't return to my homelands, to my family and my territory-specific Ceremonies. This hindered my healing process and further disenfranchised my emotional, mental, and spiritual development. Upon returning, I have found myself screaming out in reaction to violence, grief, and trauma to find that my ability to cope has increased, this energy inside of me allowed to be excised.

Through this experience I realized the importance of my own culture in relation to my health: to be able to reconnect and be held meant I could honour my body in its multitudes and shed the colonial western standards of what healing and coping look like.

Thoughts on an Anarchist Response to Hepatitis C and HIV

Alexander McClelland and Zoë Dodd

[Authors' note: We wrote this piece on anarchist responses to HIV and Hepatitis C five years ago. In some places, we have updated information in the text to reflect today's context. The words in this piece are increasingly relevant today. The drug policy crisis, ongoing HIV criminalization, and COVID-19 have ramped up all of our concerns. We have both continued our engagement toward realizing the health and well-being of our communities—working and thinking, in, against, and beyond— for transformation and emancipation. —AM and ZD, 2021]

"As a woman living with HIV, I am often asked whether there will ever be a cure for AIDS. My answer is that there is already a cure. It lies in the strength of women, families and communities, who support and empower each other to break the silence around HIV/AIDS and take control ..."
—BEATRICE WERE, UGANDAN AIDS ACTIVIST[115]

INTRODUCTION

In the early days of the HIV epidemic, within a context of massive and systemic state neglect, people who were impacted and affected by HIV came together out of desperation and urgency to help care for and support their own communities, friends, and families. This care and support took many forms. Some helped people die with dignity in nonstigmatizing environments, while others pooled medications in buyers' clubs and distributed them to one another outside of official health care systems of access. Still others established collective community clinics; developed community prevention, support, and care organizations; and distributed sterile equipment for injecting drugs, even when it was deemed illegal by the state, or opened supervised consumption sites without official institutional forms of medical or public health approval. Despite these productive examples, which undoubtedly saved many lives, the devastating past of the AIDS crisis is not one to be romanticized. This is not our intention.

In looking back at history, we can see that many of these radical actions were inherently anarchist. At the time, people's intentions may not have been rooted in an anarchist world view. People did what they needed to do to maintain their own survival despite what higher authorities deemed appropriate. These examples are the active realization of mutual aid, spontaneity, trust, and collaboration—all tenets of anarchism. While anarchism was not central to those organizing in the early days of the AIDS movement, there was an anarchist component to New York City's AIDS Coalition To Unleash Power (ACT UP) and Toronto's AIDS ACTION NOW!, and there have been many smaller anarchist AIDS activist initiatives over the years. We aim to help reconnect the work of these past movements to what is happening today, or what could happen in the future, with liberatory concepts and ideas brought forward through anarchism.

Together we have decades of experience in addressing Hepatitis C and HIV as radicals, anarchists, activists, researchers, and frontline workers. Born out of frustration, optimism, and a desire to change things, our goal is to examine ways of thinking—while intentionally engaged with an anarchist world view—to see how those most impacted by Hepatitis C and/or HIV, as well as other conditions, could merge these ideas to put the actualization of health into their own hands. We are working on an ongoing writing project to enable radicals, activists, and scholars to make links between health care responses and anarchist principles.[116] This writing project has been developed collaboratively through a series of discussions with a wide range of radicals, activists, workers, anarchists, and people living with Hepatitis C and/or HIV in Canada.

We hope, through our writing, to suggest an anarchist praxis when analyzing current responses to HIV and Hepatitis C. Specifically, we aim to examine the capitalist organization of health care, reactive forms of community-based politics, and interventions focused on homogenization and hierarchical intervention—or top-down projects of prescribed sameness and standardization. The capitalist organization of health care and the reactive position activists have been forced into has created a context in which the imaginations of many people involved in the responses to HIV and Hepatitis C have been limited to what is prescribed by funding bodies, through disciplinary forms of knowledge, or what is able to be marketized. Our work aims to stretch the imaginations of HIV and Hepatitis C responses beyond the current prevailing reality. We argue that we have the tools in place to save lives and bring these diseases to an end, but instead society is organized in ways that allow for millions of people to continue to die. Our hope is that our initial writing in this area will inspire people to rethink how and why the current systems to respond to HIV and Hepatitis C are organized the way they are. With this we aim to reconsider models of collective organizing to address these diseases.

We dedicate our ongoing work to all those who live with Hepatitis C and/or HIV and those who have died as a result of purposeful state neglect, profit-driven corporations, austerity, bureaucratic red tape, war, ongoing colonization, white supremacy, institutional violence, patriarchy, transphobia, homophobia, and punitive legal systems. We have chosen to focus this article and our ongoing writing project on HIV and Hepatitis C because of our work and personal connections to these epidemics. In addition, HIV and Hepatitis C share unique elements: both are highly stigmatized diseases that disproportionately impact marginalized and state-neglected communities, and both have emerged under neoliberalism.

THE CAPITALIST ORGANIZATION OF HEALTH CARE

"The worst enemy of a government is its own population."
—NOAM CHOMSKY, LINGUIST AND ANARCHIST[117]

We are well over thirty years into the HIV crisis, and over twenty years into the Hepatitis C epidemic. Together, Hepatitis C and HIV are the first major globalized health epidemics to emerge under the neoliberal world order. Around the world there are 350,000 to 500,000 deaths attributed to Hepatitis C, and in 2020 an estimated 690,000 [480,000 to 1,000,000] people died due to AIDS-related causes[118]— primarily impacting the world's most socially and politically marginalized peoples, including people who live in poverty, people who use drugs, women, people in prison, people of colour, gay and bisexual men, trans people, sex workers, and young people.

As a distinct form of capitalist political and social organization, neoliberalism came about in the mid-1970s and has been focused on cutting back social programs, on individualism, entrepreneurship, a reduction of the state, privatization, corporate and managerial rationality, and efficiency through competition. The managerial logic of neoliberalism has come to organize a capitalist system of health care that is deeply intertwined with profit-driven transnational corporations in which illness is now profitable. This means that the ways in which we are allowed to respond to HIV and Hepatitis C are prescribed by top-down bureaucratized institutions with the aim of making or saving money. In this system, there have been massive biomedical advances, billions of dollars "invested" in biomedical research, the development of thousands of nongovernmental organizations, specified multilateral and bilateral agencies, public-private partnerships, billion-dollar cause marketing campaigns, and multiple multimillion-dollar touring conferences to address the diseases.

Using the managerial language and logic of the corporate sector, this global HIV and Hepatitis C professionalized response can limit conceptualizations of what is possible. Including framing how knowledge and meaning are produced, where often positivist, measurable, quantifiable, and "expert" forms of knowledge are privileged to provide a professional image that is efficient and strategic within capitalism. For example, forms of social science research developed on HIV and Hepatitis C often reveal what people already know on the ground. But instead, the results come to produce a kind of expert knowledge, that, as a commodity, can be used by authorities to justify forms of hierarchical decision-making that lose sight of people's actual needs. This is the case with the current imperative to develop research "evidence" on the benefits of housing for people living with HIV and Hepatitis C in a North American context. There is even an annual touring housing- and HIV-focused conference. At this event various professionals present research, for example, on randomized control trials using forms of housing for active drug users, housing that is linked to care and also managed in close contact with the police as a method to reduce HIV infections. Here, a basic need, such as housing, becomes understood as a form of control that is used instrumentally to support public health goals. In this context, resources are diverted to expertized forms of research, with the never-ending imperative for evidence—when all that is actually needed is affordable housing.[119]

While there is no cure for HIV, since the mid-1990s, a range of drugs have been developed which can effectively block the virus from replicating and therefore keep the HIV suppressed in the body. This results in people being able to live with the virus for the full extent of their natural lives while no longer being infectious to others. Taken in combination, these drugs have been massively effective at saving people's lives—but only for those who have access. Access to these medications is governed through a system that privileges pharmaceutical company patents and profit and results in further exacerbating existing wealth disparities around the world. People continue to die regularly due to lack of access to medications that are still out of reach to the nearly 15 million people who need them.

For Hepatitis C, new treatments have shown cure rates of 90 to 100 percent with limited side effects. The pharmaceutical company Gilead Sciences earned $30 billion US between 2016 and 2020 from their new Hepatitis C treatment.[120] The drugs currently cost $1,000 US per pill per day, for a course of treatment costing a total of $84,000 US.[121] Yet, the actual cost to manufacture this new pill is estimated to be less than $250 US for the full course of treatment.[122] This treatment and others now constitute a cure for Hepatitis C, and could promise global Hepatitis C eradication. While society now has the ability to effectively cure Hepatitis C, this drug is wildly out of reach for most people due to the patenting system, cost barrier, and the capitalist profit imperative. Access to these treatments at the time of writing is extremely limited, and people are dying without access to these life-saving drugs.

THE PROBLEM OF DEFENSIVE FORMS
OF ACTIVIST STRUGGLE

Activist projects on Hepatitis C and HIV have been most often focused on defensive struggles to respond to and document the violence of governments and state institutions. For example, activist and research efforts have focused on identifying bureaucratic and legal barriers to treatment and care, or highlighting and evaluating the punitive and regressive laws, which criminalize drug users, sex workers, and people living with HIV and/or Hepatitis C. The vast majority of community organizing around Hepatitis C and HIV revolves around making claims on the state, including claims for human rights, claims for funding, and entitlements for forms of citizenship. This results in activists and community groups spending enormous amounts of time working to address administrative, institutional, bureaucratic, and legal barriers imposed by higher authorities, while at the same time reinforcing the role of the authorities they are challenging. In many cases, if they engage in activism or advocacy, community-based organizations are then put into tenuous relationships with the same authorities that provide funding for HIV and Hepatitis C programs.

In this context, social scientists, academics, and certain activist groups clamour to develop projects aiming to document or reveal the latest ways in which "key populations"(i.e., sex workers, people who use drugs, gay men, and other men who have sex with men) are being marginalized and barred access to rights and other forms of health and citizenship so that we can develop "new" evidence to help enable change. Here, the newest disastrous conservative policy or intervention becomes the newest hot research topic to dissect, consume, critique, and produce knowledge on.

Two examples of very current and necessary defensive activist struggles are the war on people who use drugs, and the criminalization of HIV exposure and nondisclosure (e.g., allegedly not telling sex partners that one is HIV-positive).

For people who use drugs, the continued rising rate of new infections of both HIV and Hepatitis C can largely be attributed to the practices of criminalization which have targeted and locked up millions of people and created devastating levels of stigma. Criminalization practices under the war on drugs actively deny people access to effective ways to have autonomy over their own lives and to reduce infections through harm reduction interventions, which include needle distribution, supervised consumption sites, and opioid substitution therapy. People who treat Hepatitis C, including doctors and specialists, regularly deny those with the disease access to treatment based on their drug use history. Although drug use is not a criterion for exclusion in the guidelines for Hepatitis C treatment in Canada, health care professionals continually deny treatment based on moral judgments about drug use, allowing people to die in the process. Although people who inject drugs make up 70 percent of new infections, only about 1 percent have received treatment in Canada.[123]

With regards to the criminalization of HIV exposure and non-disclosure, Canada is now one of the leading countries in the world to criminalize people with HIV who do not tell sex partners their HIV status, with upwards of 220 cases brought before the courts to date.[124] The application of the law in these cases is radically counter to the lived reality of HIV today, where anti-HIV medications (if available and taken by the individual) can reduce viral loads to the point where people are no longer infectious. Most often the charge applied is aggravated sexual assault, one of the harshest in the Criminal Code of Canada. This, despite the fact that in many of these cases HIV was never transmitted and the sex was consensual. For those prosecuted, the most extreme measures in the Canadian penal and policing apparatus are employed, including "offenders" being recorded on provincial and national sex offender registries and held in segregation units, including administrative segregation—solitary confinement.

We see it as vital that activists continue to fight against repressive legal structures that are out of touch with people's lived realities. But imagine what would be possible in the world if we could move beyond these legal systems of domination? In the defensive and time-consuming position of responding to these punitive practices, activists often have no time to envision what else might be possible to address these diseases in proactive and more positive ways. Alternate ways of working are hard to envision when your communities are dying, being locked up, or struggling to survive. Our focus becomes one of survival, but imagine if we did not have to engage in these oppressive struggles?

THOUGHTS ON ANARCHISM AND RESPONSES TO HIV AND HEPATITIS C

We want to be very clear that we do not expect readers to be well read in anarchist theory. Rather, we would like to highlight that there are many anarchist principles already active in our daily lives and in our communities. This is especially true of responses to Hepatitis C and HIV, where people strive and fight for equitable access to medical knowledge and life-saving medications, bodily autonomy, participation in decision-making, ensuring interventions are informed by lived experiences and grassroots knowledge, emancipation from forms of oppression, and the right to dignity and social justice for all people. Often those working in the Hepatitis C and HIV responses are not aware that the above stated goals are exactly what anarchists strive to achieve. Those who do not understand anarchist theory often equate it with violence and destruction, which is the opposite of what anarchism intends to make possible: to jointly build a noncoercive society, free of oppression and exploitation. Many people in the HIV and Hepatitis C responses already enact anarchist theories without being aware that they are anarchist.

With our approach, we aim to resist the modernist project of proposing hyperrational and universalizing forms of social organization that are rooted in a false paradigm of linear progress. We believe that theoretical forms of social organization that are *not* grounded in people's lived realities have the potential to be dangerous, oppressive, and violent. Ideology, for the purposes of our project, refers to what queer radical Gary Kinsman states as: "forms of knowledge that attends to managing people's lives that are not grounded in actual experiences and practices."[125] What we propose is what anarchist scholar James C. Scott calls a "process-oriented" anarchist view, or anarchism through the integration of theory and practice.[126] What this means is that addressing social problems must come through a dialectical relationship between concerned groups of people over time. A practical and grounded approach to anarchism ensures that we can be flexible, fluid, responsive, spontaneous, and resistant to the solely ideological.

THE VIOLENCE OF HIERARCHY AND HOMOGENIZATION

The primary way in which aspects of a capitalist society are organized is through projects of homogenization and hierarchy—or forms of top-down social planning prescribing sameness and standardization. We can see examples of these processes in settler-colonization, taxation, land ownership, urban planning, education, universal laws, and public health projects such as HIV and Hepatitis C "seek and treat" prevention as treatment initiatives. Such ideological approaches to social and political organization are often concerned with the "administration of things" through forms of centralized top-down social planning.[127] These systems often see one solution to social problems, and they produce projects of standardization that are designed to displace local, traditional, and vernacular practices with hierarchical forms of organization. They often mobilize forms of synoptic surveillance onto populations, or simultaneous forms of technological mass surveillance, that are aimed to help quantify people's lives in different ways so as to produce homogeneity and make things more rational to higher authorities. Interventions that result from these approaches can force a singular solution onto people in ways that can be disconnected from people's local knowledge of their daily lives. This singular vision of social planning is counter to an anarchist world view, which is interested in decentralization, heterogeneity, and respect for local knowledge and specificities.

The project of homogenization is also a key aspect of the Hepatitis C and HIV responses, as homogenization has been a major component of the grand modernist project of science itself, which has understood that the natural world and the human body can be made knowable, classifiable, and rational through the work of highly trained experts developing specialized forms of knowledge. One could argue that epidemic management is only possible through a top-down system of surveillance, identification, containment, regulation, and control. The centralized management and standardization of information has helped us understand the scope of the epidemics, to understand who is most impacted by the two diseases and where they are located. But if we look back in history, people have been utilizing the power of cooperation and horizontal forms of feminist organization since the beginning of the AIDS and Hepatitis C crises. But over time these ways of organizing—through forms of financial coercion such as granting systems which privilege certain forms of intervention and require bureaucracies—have been forced to change and conform to the standards of authorities, and thus, generally, we have not been able to see the realization of alternate forms of organizing in response to the two diseases.

Today in response to HIV and Hepatitis C, interventions must always be "scaled-up," official, systematized, credentialized, regulated, and organized hierarchically. For example, as governed by the United Nations, every country is supposed to have a top-down national AIDS strategy to frame how the state response is organized, so as to prescribe programs of action onto diverse local communities. Often these plans promote a singular ideological vision for how to respond to social problems without addressing or understanding the reality of those groups. Just as often, they initiate hierarchical systems of representation and participation (such as with the Country Coordinating Mechanisms of the Global Fund), which privilege the participation of representatives that speak the language—linguistically and figuratively—and follow the rules of the higher authority. In this system, local cultures, vernacular practices, and community norms are seen as barriers, or in opposition to official "effective" and "rational" Hepatitis C and HIV responses, and thus must be intervened in and changed to make people's practices acceptable to universal norms.

One of the biggest current trends in the HIV response and possibly soon to be in the Hepatitis C responses are massively funded country-wide "seek and treat" interventions. The BC Centre for "Excellence" in HIV/AIDS (quotations added) initiated this program in British Columbia, Canada, in a partnership with the medical establishment, government, and public health officials. The purpose of the program is to test populations of people deemed "at-risk" and put them on treatment. Many of these people are living in Vancouver's Downtown Eastside and are injection drug users, struggling in poverty, many without housing. In the program, if people test positive for HIV, they are immediately put on treatment so as to prevent future onward transmissions. This approach is part of what is known as "treatment as prevention." It is a new norm of HIV intervention, where people with HIV are tested as soon as possible and immediately put on treatment to reduce their viral load and thus make them less "infectious" to others. In the "seek and treat" model, HIV-testing fairs are held in public parks and there is a financial incentive to get tested. Overall, this intervention views people with HIV as vectors of disease who can be instruments in the response to HIV and who must be tested and treated with medicines so as to protect the ideological general public. This approach is driven by a form of expert medical professional paternalism, which is forced onto people, communities, organizations, and now entire countries, from a disconnected and extra-local plane of so-called "reason and science."

It is imperative that people are able to make their own decisions as to if and when they initiate treatment, since going on anti-HIV drugs is a lifelong commitment, one with many toxic side effects, and some people do not need these pills right away. Rather than people being able to make autonomous individual choices about their own health, in the "seek and treat" intervention, the agency and autonomy of people living with HIV is undermined. People living with HIV are identified, monitored, and surveilled by higher authorities, and are coerced into being neutralized via anti-HIV treatments, or they are incarcerated or quarantined (in prisons), despite the effects of these pills on their bodies. Further, as a top-down social planning initiative, the "seek and treat" type of intervention fails to address the lived realities of people who use drugs and who are living in poverty. For illicit drug users, the monitoring and surveillance of HIV treatment puts them at risk for arrest because of their drug use. For people who are homeless and/or underhoused, taking medication every day may not be possible or a priority.

CONCLUSION:
ANARCHISM FOR HEALTH

"We live in a world that must be changed to survive."
—ZACKIE ACHMAT, SOUTH AFRICAN AIDS ACTIVIST[128]

We do not believe that there is a singular solution to social problems such as Hepatitis C and HIV. As needs and conditions change for people, so must the mechanisms to address how society will function and respond. Through ongoing dialogue, reflection, and critical engagement without hierarchy or top-down decision-making, an anarchist approach aims to ensure that people's needs are met directly, and resources to address them are made available to everyone. In our ongoing work, we are deeply inspired by those actualizing their own needs and those of their communities such as the Nigerian women working as sex workers who were taken up as participants in an early 2000s HIV treatment as prevention drug trial, a trial that was ultimately deemed a failure by USAID and the pharmaceutical company Gilead. This was one of the first Truvada treatment-as-prevention trials conducted. The drug was being tested on women who were HIV-negative as a prophylaxis to prevent future HIV transmission. Nigeria is a country with a high-prevalence rate of HIV and limited treatment access for people living with the virus. In the 1990s, to allow for a wide range of development grants, the United States demanded that Nigeria implement patent protection laws in the service of pharmaceutical company interests.[129] The result has widely restricted access of people living in poverty to life-saving HIV medications. In this context, it became rational for the HIV-negative women enrolled in the USAID and Gilead Truvada drug trial to keep all the medications for themselves (for if they tested HIV-positive at a later date), or to distribute them to family members or friends living with HIV who needed them for immediate survival. This partially resulted in the drug trial being understood as a failure by Gilead and USAID. The drug trial was discontinued, as accurate results on the use of the medications could not be determined. But the women in the drug trial did what they needed to do for themselves and their communities, despite the master plan. This response helped enable access to medication in an otherwise oppressive structure. And while they may not have seen themselves as anarchists, or activists, these women worked to support each other and their community despite what a higher authority deemed appropriate or necessary. We see the actions of these women as a success and an active realization of anarchist principles and liberatory practices to support health.

A second inspirational example is the current response to the prohibitively expensive and exclusionary access to Hepatitis C medication. In many places around the world, people who are unable to access government-funded Hepatitis C treatment have come together online in chat forums and using social media to advise one another on how to legally access affordable forms of the medication directly from generic drug manufacturers or by travelling to countries where governments have negotiated for cheaper drug prices. In the spirit of HIV buyers' clubs, virtual groups of so-called "nonprofessionals" are providing health support to one another and are subverting oppressive state and corporate systems to get what they need. A course of treatment that can cost $94,000 can thus be accessed for around $1,000.[130] We see this approach to collectivity and mutual aid as central to mobilizing forms of anarchism for health.

When thinking through antihierarchical ways of doing things, our current drive to endlessly plan, research, and provide evidence for responding to HIV and Hepatitis C can easily get in the way. Thinking through an anarchist world view requires that we question the drive to intervene in others' lives, and calls on us to reflect on the power we hold in relation to others. But generally, if people have questions of specific instances—such as what would happen here? What will happen there? How would we organize?—the answer would always be local and come from communities in question without hierarchy, and without outside interference, and without outsiders trying to make profit off bodies and illnesses. There are no specific prescribed answers except that a horizontal view means trusting that people will always innovate and, through cooperation, will help each other.

Imagine for a minute what our responses to health and HIV and Hepatitis C could look like if we did not have to constantly battle against massive state, institutional, and private sector apparatuses to get access to the means for our survival. The war on drugs, harm reduction, treatment access, criminalization, citizenship status, wealth inequity—these are all issues related to hierarchical decision-making, the liberal nation-state, and the capitalist organization of society. Now imagine what we could get done if we didn't have those systems in place. If people were able to access what they needed without a higher authority. How can we work to interrogate and provide deep philosophical reflection on *how* and *why* certain regimes of truth have come to render certain forms of social organization possible, while others are rendered impossible, too optimistic or unrealistic? What would be possible if our society *was not* organized in ways that view people's bodies as a source of capital, and where illness and disease are a revenue stream for businesses, institutions, and a range of other actors?

Regrowth in Ruins

Abolitionist Dreams for Health System Transformation

Zena Sharman

Early in the process of writing this book, a friend offered me the question, "What will grow and be birthed in the ruins of old structures?" I kept returning to her question as I grappled with the strategic implications of accepting that the health system isn't broken, it's working as designed. The strategic implications of this are important because strategy helps us articulate a vision of where we want to be and guides us as we work together to create the changes necessary to get there. Accepting that the health system is working as designed has the potential to shift how we relate to this system and how we discern what changes are needed to bring us closer to the care we dream of.

I've always been fascinated by what it takes to create change, and how to move wisely in the process of envisioning and creating those changes. I've spent the past twenty years working in roles focused on changing the health system, health research practice, or health research funding, first as a student and later in strategy-focused jobs in the health research funding sector and through my work as an LGBTQ+ health advocate. Thinking about my experiences with this work made me reckon with the fact that I spent too long believing in the inevitability of these systems.

Although I knew they were constructed by people and could therefore be changed, I unconsciously worked from the assumption that the systems themselves had a kind of permanence to them.

This belief became a constraint, especially in my work as an LGBTQ+ health advocate: I was passionate about creating change and doing my part to help move the health system toward greater equity and justice, but my thinking was limited by my belief in the inevitability of the system itself. The system became both the thing I wanted to change and the frame that bounded my thinking.

Activists and scholars working toward police and prison abolition have taught me ways of thinking about system transformation that I find generative when applied to the health system. Critical Resistance defines abolition as "both a practical organizing tool and a long-term goal," one that works toward "eliminating imprisonment, policing, and surveillance and creating lasting alternatives to punishment and imprisonment."[131] Prison industrial complex abolition is a lineage grounded in the activism, organizing, and scholarship of Black, Indigenous, and people of colour and other communities disproportionately affected by mass incarceration and police violence. Abolitionists are imaginative, visionary, accountable, and judiciously pragmatic in how they call on us to dream a different world into being while actively working toward that dream in our everyday actions. They show me what it means to make a sustained commitment to transformative organizing and what can happen when you change the framework of your thinking about what's necessary or possible. Learning from abolitionists working to end and create alternatives to imprisonment, policing, and surveillance helped me break free of the limiting frame that was constraining my ability to think about what might be possible for queer and trans health and healing.

Abolitionist approaches to transforming systems differ from what I learned about health systems change in graduate school. There, my professors taught me about rigorous approaches researchers and policy-makers used to enable health systems change. We compared the historical origins, present-day structures, strengths, and pitfalls of different health systems. We studied and researched how to make those systems better, often in collaboration with people working within the health system. I learned a lot and have continued learning in the years since by putting these ideas into practice in my own work and watching others do the same.

What was missing from all this learning and practice is that no one ever encouraged me to think beyond the system that exists the way abolitionists have modelled for me. In an essay for aspiring police and prison abolitionists, abolitionist organizer and educator Mariame Kaba invites us to begin from boundless possibilities by asking, "What can we imagine for ourselves and the world?" rather than starting from "What do we have now, and how can we make it better?"[132] One of the reasons I find Kaba's guidance helpful is it invites me to shift away from framing my thinking within the boundaries and assumptions of the current system.

I believe that many of us—myself included—have grown accustomed to thinking about LGBTQ+ health care in terms of Kaba's second question, "What do we have now, and how can we make it better?" For example, there are efforts to make health care more affirming by encouraging providers to wear pronoun pins, having more inclusive intake forms, and integrating queer and trans health–related content into medical education curriculum. While I'm all for efforts to make health care feel more inclusive for our community, I feel curious about the extent to which we're stuck in a limiting way of thinking about the changes that are needed or possible—especially when considering the potential pitfalls of inclusion within the wider landscape of the medical industrial complex.

I fear too many of us are trapped in a mindset where health care that affirms our dignity and respects our humanity is positioned as the pinnacle of what queer and trans health care could look like instead of as the bare minimum we should expect for all of our care.

I understand why we might feel this way: Every queer and trans person I know has had shitty, harmful, and sometimes violent experiences in health care. These experiences, and the dynamics underpinning them, have killed people we love and they're going to keep killing them. That we've been conditioned to have such low expectations is an indictment of the system that exists. Lowering our expectations can be a survival strategy, a way to help us as we grit our teeth, raise our protective force fields, or deliberately leave our bodies to make it through a visit with a health care provider or as we navigate the system to get the care we need. Having low expectations can feel validating when things go badly, and maybe we exhale just a little on those occasions when it's not as bad as we expected. We might even feel relieved, grateful, or surprised in those rarer instances when it actually feels pretty good.

I want this book to nudge us to shift and expand our expectations of health care, to encourage queer and trans people to dream differently and demand more, beyond inclusion and reform. The harms and violence of the existing system are real and awful. I'm not trying to tell you we can simply dream our way out of the dire circumstances we're in or that the problem is in our attitudes toward health care. *The health system is the problem, not you.* If we're going to transform the conditions under which queer and trans people experience health care, we need to think differently about the system itself and practise dreaming and building beyond it.

A CONTROLLED BURN, NOT A WILDFIRE: INCREASING THE POSSIBILITY OF FREEDOM

If you're a systems change nerd like me, you might've come across something called the adaptive cycle. It's a figure eight–shaped loop that draws on learnings from living systems like forests to help us figure out where a system (or parts of a system) is in its life cycle: Is it new and growing rapidly; mature, stable, and possibly rigid; in a state of crisis and collapse; or in a period of recovery, creativity, and change? Noticing where a system is now can help us imagine where we want it to be and develop strategies for getting there. When I get really mad or frustrated with the health system, I sometimes feel an urge to shout, "Let's burn it all down!" Tools like the adaptive cycle help me remember where to point my energy: we need a precise and controlled burn, not a wildfire that indiscriminately destroys everything in its path.

At the core of this book is the idea that we need to transform the existing health system in order to create more widespread access to liberatory health care for all LGBTQ+ people. Some institutions and systems—here I'm thinking of policing and the prison industrial complex, for example—are fundamentally harmful and violent and demand complete abolition for communities to flourish. It would be better for overall health and health equity if we were to abolish police and prisons and reinvest the vast sums we currently spend on them into housing, income supports, education, health care, food justice, environmental justice, and anything else communities need to feel healthy, connected, and safe.

The health system necessitates a different approach, one that retains elements of the current system and abolishes others, while also seeking to transform and build beyond that system. Part of our work is discerning what to keep, what to change, what to get rid of altogether, and where we want to create something new or entirely outside the system. While I'm an abolitionist when it comes to prisons and police, my stance isn't to abolish the health system, though I can understand why some people might feel this way.

My resistance to this idea might reflect the current limitations of my own imagination (and potentially my embeddedness in a place with a publicly funded health system). Still, when I think about people like my friend who's alive and well because they recently received state-of-the-art cancer treatment, I notice I don't feel ready to chuck the entire health system out the window. In an interview for the book *Prison by Any Other Name*, trans activist and mental health provider Sadie Ryanne Baker applies an abolitionist lens to the mental health care system that I think is applicable to the health system as a whole:

> "I believe we need to smash the mental health system as much as any other power structure," [Baker] says. "But, unlike systems like prison and policing, we should pick up some of the pieces and rebuild a new system with them. We must examine every individual part of the mental health care system critically by asking: 'Does this specific thing help or hurt oppressed people?'"[133]

When thinking about the kinds of changes we want to create and the system we want to build, it can be helpful to distinguish between reformist and nonreformist reforms. Migrant justice advocate Harsha Walia speaks to the kind of discernment needed when making this distinction:

> Arguably every reform entrenches the power of the state because it gives the state the power to implement that reform. But from an ethical orientation towards emancipation, I think a guiding question on non-reformist reforms is: Is it increasing the possibility of freedom?[134]

Asking ourselves, "Is it increasing the possibility of freedom?" can help us decide what changes we want to work toward and which ones to avoid, even if they might seem helpful on the surface. Transformative change takes time, so we need to take the long view, considering both the immediate and longer-term implications of potential changes. Here we can learn from abolitionist organization Critical Resistance, who are in a practice of asking, "Will we regret this in ten years?"[135]

To help make these ideas more concrete, I'll share a couple of examples of recent health-related reforms that might seem liberatory on the surface but actually are harmful to oppressed people. First is the idea of having social workers work alongside the police or replacing the police with social workers. This idea garnered popular attention in 2020 in the context of calls to defund and abolish the police galvanized by uprisings against police murders of Black, Indigenous, and people of colour, many of whom are Mad and/or disabled. Some of these murders happened in the context of people experiencing a mental health crisis or during a so-called police "wellness check," like in the cases of Regis Korchinski-Paquet, a Black Indigenous woman, and those of Chantel Moore and Renee Davis, both Indigenous women.

While on the surface, social workers might seem like a kinder, gentler alternative to the cops, abolitionist social workers Cameron Rasmussen and Kirk "Jae" James challenge this proposal on the basis of the inherent carcerality of social work. As they put it, "Social workers have a long and troubled history as partners to the state, more often serving as carceral enforcers than as collaborators toward liberation."[136] Queer, disabled, autistic, and mentally ill community organizer Stefanie Lyn Kaufman-Mthimkhulu echoes these concerns, citing examples like social workers' roles in racist patterns of child apprehension. They instead call for greater investments in peer support, including support for peer-led mobile crisis response teams.[137]

A second example is the recent proliferation of US-based queer and trans–led, for-profit, venture capital–backed LGBTQ+ health services and apps. Collectively, companies like Folx Health, Plume, and Euphoria have raised tens of millions of dollars from venture capital firms who see potential profit in their business models—"a multibillion-dollar market opportunity," in the words of one Folx investor.[138] Company founders reference their own lived experiences when speaking about the discrimination and barriers to care queer and trans people face when accessing health care. Folx and Plume promise affirming health care on queer and trans people's terms, without judgment, ignorance, or hassle, while apps like Euphoria aim to provide a technological solution to the challenges of gender transition.

Health care companies like Folx and Plume deliver slickly branded virtual services intended to make care more accessible to paying customers who might not have convenient access to affirming care close to home. While on the surface this might seem beneficial, the privatization of care further entrenches disparities in affordability and access to care. Put simply, the only people who can benefit from these privatized services are people who can afford to pay, and this excludes a huge swath of the LGBTQ+ community. A big focus of these companies' business models is gender-affirming health care like access to hormones or support letters for surgeries, all for a fee. Given higher rates of poverty among trans people—particularly those who are racialized, disabled, and/or young—these kinds of private subscription services are likely to benefit only more privileged members of the trans community, which could exacerbate disparities among trans people.[139] As trans journalist Niko Stratis wrote in an article on this phenomenon, these startups are "a neoliberal response to a crisis that capitalism doesn't have an answer for."[140] She calls for free, safe, and accessible health care for everyone who needs it.

I find it energizing to engage with questions from abolitionists in thinking through these and other possible reforms because they invite us into a different perspective on the world around us and the world we are striving to build:

What can we imagine for ourselves and the world?

Does this specific thing help or hurt oppressed people?

Is it increasing the possibility of freedom?

Will we regret this in ten years?

I want these to be the kinds of questions we engage with when thinking about LGBTQ+ health and working toward health system transformation.

WE ALREADY KNOW HOW TO DO THIS: LIBERATORY LINEAGES AND ONGOING RESISTANCE

The prospect of working to transform or replace most or all of a large, complex system can feel daunting and impossible in this lifetime, yet I take comfort in knowing communities like ours have been doing this for generations. Queer and trans people are adept at doing the prefigurative work of creating the world we want to live in through our actions today while also building toward longer-term systemic transformation. I'll bet many of you are already doing this work, even if you don't necessarily think of it this way.

The LGBTQ+ community has a long history of creativity, resistance, and mutual aid when it comes to our health and survival. We are skilled at dreaming, building, and mobilizing around health and healing, as are other communities resisting and responding to the health impacts of systemic oppression. This work happens both within and outside the existing health system. What it holds in common is a willingness to imagine something different, challenge the status quo, and experiment by doing.

Here, I share some examples of what this practice has looked like in different communities over time. There's too vast a history and a rich tapestry of present-day practices to offer a comprehensive overview. Rather, my intention is to seed our dreams of alternatives to the existing system with examples of how people and communities have resisted, created alternatives to the health system, and fostered collective healing for generations.

In the book *Before AIDS: Gay Health Politics in the 1970s*, historian Katie Batza documents the creation and evolution in the 1970s of a "largely self-sufficient gay medical system that challenged, collaborated with, and educated mainstream health practitioners."[141] By the beginning of the 1980s, this network grew to include community clinics, outreach programs, national professional organizations, and research infrastructure. It developed during an era when health and health care were explicit parts of many political projects, whether among revolutionary groups like the Black Panthers and the Young Lords or within the women's health and disability rights movements.

Batza looks at the development of this gay health network in the 1970s, focusing primarily on clinics in Boston, Chicago, and Los Angeles. At each of the clinics described in Batza's book, variously configured coalitions of community members, health care providers, medical students, and researchers worked together to organize and deliver care. In Chicago, for example, the Howard Brown Health Center grew out of a gay medical student's frustration with his school's failure to prepare him to meet his community's health needs. In response, this man—David Ostrow—created a support group for gay medical students experiencing homophobia in medical school. In 1973, Ostrow placed an ad in the *Chicago Gay Crusader*, the local gay newspaper, with a phone number other gay medical students could call to join the group. His phone rang off the hook with calls from gay medical students and people from the gay community wanting to know where they could find good, respectful, nonjudgmental health care.[142]

By 1974, Ostrow and the collaborators he met through the support group, including nurses, physicians, and medical technicians, began exploring the idea of offering medical services to the gay community, an idea that eventually grew into a community clinic. They also worked in collaboration with local bars and bathhouses to bring sexual health services directly to the community through the "VD van," a motorhome retrofitted into a mobile STI clinic where people could get tested and snack on cookies and milk. A well-known local drag queen—Nurse Wanda Lust—travelled with the van dressed in a short, tight nurse's uniform, a bright red wig, high heels, a nurse's hat, and a hairnet. She also would sometimes visit sick patients at the hospital.

Batza doesn't romanticize the history of this gay medical system, pointing to a failure to deliver "race- and feminist-conscious gay health services" and to models of care that centred cis white gay men.[143] She also describes the challenges clinics faced in navigating the wider political context of doing this work within an antiqueer assimilationist state and the compromises inherent in the formalization and nonprofitization of community care. Still, I found Batza's book fascinating because it revealed to me a history of a rich network of community-led health care I hadn't previously known about.

During the same era, revolutionary groups like the Black Panthers and the Young Lords made health an explicit part of their resistance and community organizing. In the book *Body and Soul*, Alondra Nelson documents the Black Panthers' politicized, community-centred work in health care.[144] Nelson characterizes the Black Panthers' work in this domain as "social health," which she describes as "an outlook on well-being that scaled from the individual, corporeal body to the body politic in such a way that therapeutic matters were inextricably articulated to social justice ones."[145] The Black Panthers' mission of serving the people body and soul included the creation of People's Free Medical Clinics in thirteen cities across the United States. They tested people for hypertension and lead poisoning, did testing and advocacy around sickle cell disease (which disproportionately affects Black people), trained community health workers, and offered a free breakfast program for children.

Like the Black Panthers, Puerto Rican group the Young Lords also engaged in community health activism.[146] They liberated a city-owned X-ray truck to screen community members for tuberculosis after the Tuberculosis Society repeatedly denied their requests to use it. They also tested children for lead poisoning after several died due to an epidemic of such poisoning in their community. The Young Lords occupied Lincoln Hospital in the South Bronx—known locally as "the Butcher Shop"—because of the deplorable care it provided to Latinx and Black people. Working in coalition with health care workers, the Young Lords drafted the first patient bill of rights and established the first acupuncture drug treatment centre in the United States.

In tracing lineages of health activism and community-led health care, it's important to recognize trans resistance to medical gatekeeping and how trans communities share knowledge and care for each other. Historian Jules Gill-Peterson has researched the history of trans do-it-yourself (DIY), which she describes as "an important historical home for trans knowledge and practice since the mid-twentieth century."[147] She cites the example of Edith Ferguson, a trans woman from Long Beach, California, who published a short-lived newsletter, *Transvestia*, in the early 1950s. In it, she actively critiqued the medical model of transition just as it was coming into being. Beginning in 1951, Ferguson advertised in magazines for an eighteen-month correspondence course in what she then referred to as "female impersonation." Gill-Peterson positions Ferguson's course as a form of trans DIY, one deliberately in opposition to the medical model of transition then gaining prominence.[148]

This practice of trans DIY and community knowledge-sharing has taken many forms over the years, far more than can be summarized here. I think of examples like Lou Sullivan's 1985 book *Information for the Female-to-Male Crossdresser and Transsexual*, a handbook explaining how one's body might react to hormone therapy and offering tips for FTMs on passing as men. In Canada, trans activist Rupert Raj founded several trans organizations and publications, including *Gender Review: The FACTual Journal* (1978–81).[149] There, readers could find stories written by trans community members on a range of topics including hair removal, surgery, and what a relationship between a doctor and a trans patient should look like.[150]

I'm reminded of Cooper Lee Bombardier's story of learning to self-inject testosterone from a friend, an older trans man who used to buy hormones in Mexico in the late 1980s and carry them across the border. As Bombardier writes, "My friend was my teacher, because seventeen years ago, that's what we had. Just each other."[151] micha cárdenas writes similarly of learning from other trans women in a private social media group about self-managing her hormones to make gametes when she was trying to conceive a baby. She describes her experiences in poetry:

> Other trans women taught me how to do it.
> Sadie said, get a microscope,
> don't pay hundreds of dollars for doctor visits to check your semen,
> with a $50 kids microscope,
> you can see sperm,
> morphology and motility.[152]

I adore this story for how it speaks to trans women's brilliance, creativity, and DIY reclamations of science and medicine. It reminds me of the GynePunks, a Barcelona-based group of queer and trans radical bio-hackers and TransHackFeminists who have created DIY tools (a centrifuge, a microscope, and an incubator) for analyzing body fluids and a 3-D printable speculum.[153] They freely share instructions for building these tools as well as how to use them for self-examination and testing. Their work intentionally rejects and resists the anti-Black racism, sexism, and violence so central to the history of modern gynecology.[154]

In my own community, there's the Catherine White Holman Wellness Centre (CWHWC), a volunteer-run, low-barrier wellness centre by and for trans and gender-diverse people. The CWHWC was founded by nurse practitioner Fin Gareau, a trans, Indigenous Two-Spirit person, as his nursing school practicum project. Over ten years later, the CWHWC continues to offer free counselling and legal services to people regardless of citizenship, health insurance, or residential address. The Centre purposefully exists outside the formal health system so as to retain greater community control and autonomy over how care is delivered.

I've also seen change happen at a whole system level in my home province through the leadership and sustained efforts of trans and queer people working inside the formal health system. Their work led to the development of Trans Care BC, a province-wide program created in 2015 to enhance and coordinate trans health services and supports across the British Columbia.[155] Among their accomplishments is the 2019 opening of the BC-based Gender Surgery Program, the only publicly funded clinic providing gender-affirming lower surgeries in Western Canada.[156] Before this, trans people who wanted these surgeries had to travel over 4,500 kilometres to Montreal, where they lacked access to their communities and support networks as well as dealing with the extra costs of travel and pain of flying cross-country not long after surgery.

Trans Care has increased access to publicly funded gender-affirming upper surgeries by working to grow the number of qualified surgeons in the province from three to fifteen. They offer a range of other services, too, like helping people with health system navigation, supporting peer and community groups across the province, and creating educational resources and training for health care providers.

Another health system–based example worth noting is Casa de Salud, an integrative primary care centre in Albuquerque, New Mexico. It offers a model of care rooted in cultural humility, community organizing, and low-barrier, dignified access to health care. Founded in 2004, they provide low-cost primary care, acute care, counselling/therapy, acupuncture, massage, reiki, curanderismo, and Indigenous-based healing circles. Casa de Salud works to "center and uplift marginalized communities," which they describe as "those who either have been traditionally othered by the health care system (immigrants, monolingual Spanish speaking patients, LGBT/queer community members, and community members struggling with addictions)."[157] Their work integrates a harm reduction approach; alongside their other services, they operate a syringe exchange, offer training in reversing overdoses, and provide access to integrative, community-based models of addiction treatment for people seeking this kind of care.

Their executive director is Anjali Taneja, a queer family physician, organizer, and DJ whose work on the medical industrial complex is discussed in the chapter called "The System Isn't Broken, It's Working as Designed." As of 2018, a third of Casa de Salud's staff identified as LGBTQ+ and 50 percent identified as people of colour.[158] They also have a Health Apprentice program that trains community members in primary care, "from triage and charting to injections, blood draws and many other treatments," alongside training in anti-racism and cultural humility.[159] Many of these volunteers go on to careers in health care; in a 2021 interview, Taneja noted that in 2015, 10 percent of the incoming class of medical students at the University of New Mexico were former Health Apprentices.[160]

Currently, around 75 to 80 percent of Casa de Salud's patients are uninsured and the remainder are on Medicaid.[161] For patients who can afford to pay, visits cost forty dollars and payment is optional. The centre has intentionally chosen a nonprofit model in which their funding comes from a mix of community, foundations, and county and state contracts.[162] In describing their model, Taneja differentiates it from a free clinic model where they "would be dependent on rich white people to make it function."[163] Rather, they're focused on building power with their community, including by helping individual patients to decrease their medical debts—by over $2.5 million to date—as well by engaging in advocacy through building a patient coalition focused on addressing the drivers of this debt.

Learning from abolition is a theme running through this chapter, and some health care providers are explicitly working with abolitionist politics within the health system. For example, in Canada a collective of health care workers, lawyers, advocates, community organizers, and frontline care providers working with people who've experienced incarceration recently created the *Caring for People Who Are Detained* zine. It's a resource for frontline care providers to engage with abolitionist practices and minimize harms when their patients are detained or accompanied by law enforcement.[164] In it, they offer practical advice for providers, like how to document injuries patients may have suffered at the hands of police and how to interview patients when cops are present. They also offer strategies for planning patient aftercare given the abhorrent lack of health care people will likely face once incarcerated in a jail, prison, or detention centre.

In Oakland, California, health care workers are organizing with their communities to help people find alternatives to calling 911 during health emergencies. The Oakland Power Projects (OPP) was founded by Critical Resistance in 2015 as part of their fight to end the use of imprisonment, policing, and surveillance as responses to social, economic, and political problems. In response to calls from community members to disconnect health crises and healing from police response, OPP convened an Anti-Policing Healthworkers Cohort made up of emergency medical technicians, free clinic workers, emergency room doctors, nurses, acupuncturists, and herbalists. Together, they began offering workshops designed to empower communities to access health care without involving law enforcement. The workshops focused on acute emergencies, behavioural health, and overdose prevention; they trained community members on things like how to deal with gunshot wounds, intervene in mental health crises, and reverse overdoses, all without calling 911. Their learnings and curriculum are summarized in an Anti-Policing Health Toolkit.[165]

In Sacramento and Oakland, organizers with the Anti Police-Terror Project launched Mental Health First (MH First) in 2020, a model of nonpolice responses to mental health crises. MH First currently offers services by phone or text message on weekend nights when other mental health services aren't available. If someone is experiencing a psychiatric emergency, needs substance use support, or is in a domestic violence situation they need help getting out of, they can contact MH First. Their intention is to "interrupt and eliminate the need for law enforcement in mental health crisis first response by providing mobile peer support, de-escalation assistance, and non-punitive and life-affirming interventions."[166] Their model is rooted in decriminalization, decreasing stigma, and addressing the root causes of violence and harm: white supremacy, capitalism, and colonialism. MH First cofounder Cat Brooks contrasts their focus on "time, de-escalation, compassion, and care"—which might involve being on the phone with someone for hours—with how law enforcement tends to want to "deal with these, which usually requires force or incarceration."[167]

MH First program director Asantewaa Boykin, who also cofounded the Anti Police-Terror Project, is an emergency room nurse. Boykin describes MH First's approach as "self-determined crisis management." Their goal is to "get you from where you are to your next step. And not to tell you what that step is, but to help you determine what that step is."[168] It's a model rooted in relationships and meeting people where they're at. That might look like helping someone make a safety and mental health plan, figuring out how to change their current situation in a way that works for them, or planning a follow-up call with an MH First volunteer. In non-COVID times, it might also look like dispatching a team made up of a mental health professional, a registered nurse, or emergency medical technician, and a security liaison whose job it is to manage the presence of community members and law enforcement.[169]

Sex workers and people who use drugs have long been innovative creators and practitioners of community-led health care and harm reduction. In Chicago, for example, the Young Women's Empowerment Project (YWEP)—an organization by and for young people of colour with current or former experience in the sex trade and street economies—ran a youth-led syringe exchange for a decade. In an interview, former YWEP director Shira Hassan described their work as "trying to figure out solutions for staying alive and having each other's backs."[170] As described elsewhere in this book (see the interview with Anita "Durt" O'Shea), there's also San Francisco's St. James Infirmary, a health clinic by and for sex workers that's been running for over twenty years.

In an article chronicling anarchist responses to the overdose crisis, Zoë Dodd and Alexander McClelland describe different strategies activists have used to reduce the harms of laws and policies that criminalize drugs and the people who use them.[171] They cite the example of harm reduction workers who found ways to bring Naloxone—a medication used to counteract overdoses—into Canada and train others to use it at a time when it was only available via prescription. They also tell the story of the Crack Pipe Train, an underground network of drug users and allies in Toronto who helped distribute crack pipes to drug users in Montreal when these supplies were not yet being made available by the city's public health officials. They point to efforts by workers within health and social services to resist state surveillance and collection of data about people who use drugs. These databases are used to collect information on people's health history and drug use, often without their informed consent, and their data can be shared with health care providers, social workers, and others. Workers resisted by inputting minimal information, no information, or anonymized information that can't be linked to a specific person.

Indigenous people and communities have long-standing practices of organizing around health and healing as a form of resistance against the ongoing impacts of colonization. One example is the Native Youth Sexual Health Network (NYSHN). NYSHN was created by a group of Indigenous youth in 2008 and has since "grown into a grassroots network of Indigenous youth leaders across Turtle Island, working to respond to the sexual and reproductive health, rights and justice needs of [their] communities."[172] Collectively led by and for Indigenous youth under thirty, NYSHN is advised by three councils: the National Indigenous Young Women's Council, the National Indigenous Youth Council on HIV/AIDS, and the National Native American Youth Council on HIV/AIDS.[173] NYSHN's youth leaders are supported by a network of aunties and mentors.

One of NYSHN's recent projects is *You Are Made of Medicine*, a mental health peer support manual written by and for Indigiqueer, Two-Spirit, LGBTQ+, and gender-diverse Indigenous youth.[174] It explores topics like the connections between colonialism and trauma and knowing your rights when accessing mental health supports, as well as offering tools like a safety-planning worksheet and information on herbal supports for depression and anxiety. Another of NYSHN's key areas of work focuses on Indigenizing harm reduction, grounded in a four-fire model that centres sovereignty, cultural safety, reclamation, and self-determination.[175]

NYSHN hosts Sexy Health Carnivals at the invitation of Indigenous communities. The carnival was originally created by NYSHN Youth Facilitator Alexa Lesperance with the help of her community, Naotkamegwanning First Nation, as a way of breaking "barriers of fear, stigma and shame" around topics like suicide, harm reduction, consent, sexual violence prevention, sexually transmitted infections, birth control, and masturbation.[176] The carnivals feature games, prizes, safer sex supplies, and culturally safe health information. You can learn more about them in NYSHN's *Sexy Health Carnival Toolkit*, created by and for Indigenous youth.[177]

Another core area of NYSHN's work focuses on "the impacts of environmental violence including extractive industries (i.e., mining, gas, oil, logging)" on Indigenous sexual and reproductive health, rights, and justice.[178] They do frontline work with communities, and also undertake projects like *Violence on the Lands, Violence on Our Bodies*. This multi-year project, done in partnership with the Women's Earth Alliance, documented how extractive industries affect the sexual and reproductive health of Indigenous women, Two-Spirit people, and young people in North America and developed a tool kit to support them in resisting environmental violence in their communities.[179]

Also working in the areas of Indigenous health and reproductive justice is the ekw'í7tl doula collective, a Vancouver-based network of Indigenous doulas and student midwives. The collective was cofounded in 2015 and serves families who self-identify as Indigenous. They care for clients who are "racialized Indigenous and Indigenous LGBTQ2 people, people who use drugs, people involved with child welfare, insecurely housed folks," and people who have travelled to Vancouver from rural, remote, or northern communities to access pregnancy and birthing care.[180] In some Indigenous communities, pregnant people are unable to give birth in their home communities because they lack access to the health care that would enable them to do so. This is a manifestation of colonial medical violence that disrupts sacred cycles of birthing in Indigenous peoples' traditional territories.

In an interview with ekw'í7tl doula collective member Danette Jubinville, who is of Cree, Saulteaux, Jewish, and mixed-European ancestry, she describes how residential schools and the project of colonization "really targeted [Indigenous] families and the relationships between parents and their children," which has profound, violent, and intergenerational impacts.[181] Reclaiming Indigenous birthing traditions and parenting methods is an integral part of Indigenous cultural resurgence. That's why ekw'í7tl developed an Indigenous doula training workshop first offered in 2019. The curriculum centres Indigenous methodologies and ways of knowing and includes "an Indigenous reproductive justice framework for understanding how colonialism has impacted Indigenous experiences in reproductive health."[182] Roberta Williams, a doula from the Gwa'sala-'Nakwaxda'xw Nations who participated in the training, later attended the birth of the first child born in Kwagu'ł territory in over thirty years. In an interview about the experience, Williams said, "To have a birth in your traditional territory was so surreal … I can tell our ancestors were watching over smiling."[183]

Disabled people often cultivate sophisticated grassroots networks of knowledge sharing and community care where they share tips, medications, equipment, and medical advocacy tips. Disabled activists have also been leaders in mobilizations against state and health system policies and practices that threaten disabled people's lives. In 2019, disability justice activist and organizer Stacey Park Milbern worked with other disabled people to organize #PowerToLive, a grassroots campaign in response to power shutdowns causing nearly a million households in Northern California to lose electrical power. These kinds of shutdowns could have a huge impact on disabled people who use electricity-powered devices like ventilators, CPAP machines, and wheelchairs to live. The mutual aid–based #PowerToLive campaign included an online form people could use to request and offer assistance, as well as a crowdsourced survival guide for making it through these kinds of power shutdowns. Their guide included everything from "tips for keeping insulin and other temperature-sensitive medications cool, to a rundown of different kinds of in-home generators and batteries to choose from and the hourly wattage required to power different types of devices."[184]

During the COVID-19 pandemic, disabled and fat activists worked alongside others to mobilize resistance against discriminatory triage protocols and vaccine access through the #NoBodyIsDisposable campaign.[185] They fought back against medical care rationing practices that position disabled people, fat people, older people, and people with HIV/AIDS or other illnesses as less worthy of access to life-saving or life-sustaining medical care. They created know-your-rights guides for people to use when accessing health care and did media and political advocacy. They also created and shared tools for people to use in advocating for prioritizing vaccine access for older adults, disabled people, and fat people, especially those who are Indigenous, Black, Latinx, or Asian.

CARE AS RESISTANCE, RISK AS SURVIVAL

What I've shared here are among a long list of examples of different ways communities have taken up the fight for their own health and organized to create access to the kinds of care they want and need— the care they dream of. Think of what I've shared as a collection of possibilities, not an exhaustive chronicle. No list could ever be complete because this work is growing, changing, and adapting all the time as people work toward health and healing as part of larger liberatory projects and the everyday work of community care.

As I think about my own abolitionist dreams for health system transformation, I remember Robyn Maynard's words: "The opposite of a carceral state is a care-based society."[186] Maynard situates her work within a Black feminist project of care, one that challenges the anti-Black racism inherent in whose lives are deemed disposable and who is perceived as worthy of care. When I reflect on the examples shared in the latter part of this chapter, I think about how they're threaded together by care, resistance, imagination, and a tenacious commitment to doing the work needed to support people and communities to survive and flourish in the face of all the forces that seek to diminish or destroy them.

This sometimes means taking actions to reduce the harms of the system that exists, while recognizing these tactics can't fundamentally alter or destroy the oppressive systems we currently live within. It also means taking risks and taking action. In this spirit, Zoë Dodd and Alexander McClelland describe risk-taking as a path to survival:

> We are in a position where our only path to survival is to bypass state imposed red tape, rules and regulations. To help our friends, families and ourselves, it is our ethical responsibility to take things into our own hands. We must undermine the barriers enforced by bureaucratic hierarchies. We must take risks, and we must act.[187]

Close your eyes. Think: What are the risks you've taken to save your own life and your communities'? How did it feel? What worked? What was scary or didn't work? What are the risks you haven't taken yet, that you might want to dare to take to save your communities now? As we dream new forms of care into being, may we do so with a spirit of resistance, creativity, and mutual aid, from a place of courage and boundless possibilities.

Putting Yourself on the Line

Interview with Ronica Mukerjee

Ronica Mukerjee, MSN, DNP, FNP-BC, MsA, LAc, AAHIVS, is a family nurse practitioner, acupuncturist, and psychiatric mental health nurse practitioner (in training), as well as the creator and coordinator of the Gender and Sexuality Health Justice program at the Yale University School of Nursing. They specialize in care for LGBTQ+ communities, people using injection and other drugs, and people who are HIV-positive. They are a founding member and codirector of Refugee Health Alliance, a volunteer-led LGBTQ+-inclusive refugee and migrant health care clinic with soup kitchen and free potable water fountain located in Tijuana, Mexico. Ronica coedited the book *Clinician's Guide to LGBTQIA+ Care: Cultural Safety and Social Justice in Primary, Sexual, and Reproductive Healthcare*. Our conversation underscores how borders are an LGBTQ+ health issue and is a call to action for health care providers to put themselves on the line for liberation.

Zena: Part of your nursing practice involves working with communities in Mexico, close to the border with the United States. What has this experience taught you about the ways borders are a threat to people's health? Why is it important to think about the violence of borders in relation to queer and trans health?

Ronica: Borders are easy to ignore, yet they function as barriers wherein the least privileged people can be stopped from accessing resources on the other, more privileged side. LGBTQ+ people are often among the least privileged of any group of people who have access to the least resources, in this case migrants to the US-Mexico border. I've been working for more than two years at this border and I can say with a lot of confidence that tens of thousands of LGBTQ+ people have come here in the last couple of years searching for a place where they could experience greater acceptance, and although they are hoping it will be the United States, they are often rejected or not even considered for asylum, a process that is inaccessible and unaffordable for many people.

The border is not a safe place for people who are queer and trans. There are so many people who have created an industry around queer and trans border bodies, through underpaid sex work jobs (because poor queer and trans sex workers generally make less money) and poorly paid labour jobs like factory-floor positions. These jobs too often harm people's bodies before they even cross and then are shoved into detention, or most recently, rejected again and again or deported if they manage to get across in a way that is unsanctioned.

It is crucial that queer and trans North Americans be aware of the ways borders throw people away and exploit many kinds of people including queer and trans Black and Brown migrants. We see increased rates of HIV acquisition, sexually transmitted infections (STIs), physical trauma symptoms, post-traumatic stress disorder (PTSD), depression, anxiety, schizoaffective disorders, diabetes, hypertension, and many untreated, highly curable diseases at the border, caused or worsened by all of the issues and structural conditions that force people to the borders.

People barely survive their border experiences and queer and trans Americans and Canadians need to know that.

Borders that serve as various types of checkpoints, like the US-Mexico border or Israel-Palestine or India-Kashmir-Pakistan, are murderous, exploitative, artificial places and undoubtedly one of the biggest barriers to health in the world. We should not ignore their impact because we as Americans and Canadians benefit from the cheap labour that happens there. This is a crucial part of the intrinsic violence of borders, the advantage for the privileged that is derived from their pathological existence.

The United States, for example, has a very clear relationship to the Mexican border, which is a conduit for cheap goods including many of our steel-based goods, food, and drugs. Cheap goods always mean exploitation. In this case, the ones experiencing this exploitation are migrants and Mexicans on the other side of the border. People die or spend most of their lives in factories, mines, and farms for Americans to have cheap goods, but those same people are not welcome within us borders.

Zena: What have you had to learn—or unlearn—in your nursing practice in order to provide health care in ways that feel aligned with your values and political commitments? How has this shaped your practice? How has it shaped your work as a nurse educator?

Ronica: A big part of what I've had to unlearn is what a "healthy" patient looks like. There is a primacy about health, healthy bodies, and healthy communities in health care that really needs to be rejected. Very few people fall into those categories. How many people do you know who would say, "I'm a completely healthy person"? And why can't we be healthy while we're using drugs, or diabetic, or fat, or neurodivergent, or in a wheelchair? Why aren't those considered to be healthy bodies and minds, too? I've had to unlearn the narrow view of health I was taught, because a big part of health care is to imagine a "healthy" body as one that is white, cishet, nondisabled, thin, and young.

Often, when we say "healthy," one of the things we're implicitly communicating is, is this person worthy? Are they worth being alive? Health care often tries to take ownership of people's health journeys in a way that's completely false. It's not helpful to the patient or for greater understanding of the communities we're serving.

Although I rarely use this terminology when I talk to patients, part of my job is to help them reframe themselves in terms of what they've learned a healthy person is, so that they are included in this vision in a way that makes sense for them.

There are so many times when my patients will come in and they'll be like, "I fucked up and I used heroin twice in the last week" and I'll say to them, "Okay, why did that happen? Was there a trigger or something that happened?" And then their trigger will be so intense that I'm like, "I can't believe you only used heroin twice in the last week! It's amazing you knew the way you needed to cope and did it because not everyone is capable of doing that."

In health care, we don't pay enough attention to the cumulative effects of chronic stress (allostatic load) on people's health. We don't talk about microaggressions, being kicked out of your home by your parents, societal rejection, or what it's like to live in a place where political leaders are trying to legislate you out of existence. "Resilience" is a troubling word, but if we're going to talk about it as a thing, we need to know what it is for everyone; not everyone is under constant, unending attack and trying to emotionally and otherwise grow from there. I would say pretty much all my patients have PTSD and that's where I'm working from. It's inherently biased to say some people are resilient and some people aren't.

Health care providers ought to give people health advice that fits with the people who have the least resources, not the people who have the most. Do you have access to fresh fruits and vegetables and a place to safely store and cook food? Do you have the capacity to get somewhere where you can exercise in a way that's accessible to you?

When we assume every person has access to the same resources middle-class white people have, we exclude a lot of people. We can always ask our patients to be more involved in their health care. But I think that also requires us to know what they can and can't do, what they have access to and what matters most to them when it comes to their health.

Zena: How do the principles of harm reduction inform your nursing practice and the care you provide to LGBTQ+ folks?

Ronica: Harm reduction is about the model of health care you provide. But it's also about divestment from capitalism, imperialism, and prisons. It's about not calling the police, including in clinical settings where we are often taught to see them as our allies. It's about understanding that the people whose bodies get treated the worst are the ones we need to give extra time and care to.

Harm reduction is about disability justice. Our patients with disabilities often don't have access to a lot of health care facilities. Increasing people's ability to function as much as they want to in their bodies and decreasing the harms they experience should be part of our goals as care providers. We're all temporarily able-bodied and we need to start acknowledging this better and more.

We need to value what labour looks like for people. This includes understanding that it's unhelpful to tell our patients they have to quit their factory job or doing sex work or selling churros on the street because this is not a viable option for most people. Yet this is what providers tell their patients to do. They'll say to a patient who's working a manual job that's giving them back pain, "You have to stop doing this job," which to me absolutely creates harm and becomes an obstacle to care.

When health care providers say things like this to our patients, they have to come back to us and say, "No, I didn't quit my job or stop doing sex work." This can lead to a potentially castigating conversation with their provider and make it even harder for them to experience optimal well-being and functionality in the context of their lives. It's a form of harm reduction to understand our patients' stories and what they need to feel healthy and functional.

Practising harm reduction as a health care provider includes doing activism. By activism, I mean challenging the systemic barriers our patients face. We have to challenge the providers, institutions, and governments who create barriers to health care for our patients.

For example, although I'm not a huge policy person, challenging policy has been an important part of my career because it decreases harm. I believe I'm creating harm if I'm not challenging policies that get in the way of things like trans people accessing gender-affirming surgeries and hormones, or refugees getting asylum or preventing deportation. If I'm not part of challenging the lack of access people have, it's not as powerful as a health care intervention. Our job as health care providers isn't just to pull people out of the river of harm; our job is also to work to eliminate that river.

Zena: How do you practise solidarity with the people and communities you care for?

Ronica: I do this in two ways: One is just showing up, doing a good job, and not expecting anyone to thank me because I provide a service. I think of myself as part of an ecosystem of people that includes people living on the street and people living in homes. It includes the other providers, volunteers, and staff I work with and also how I'm situated in the communities I'm part of.

Each person has a role to play, and our roles may shift over time. At some point I may be the person who's living on the street and hopefully somebody else will take my position as a care provider. Health care providers also need to strategically distribute resources to people who tend to get them the least. We need to be insistent and willing to stand up for bodies that are not our own and don't look like our own.

The second way I practise solidarity is by understanding the science *and* what's lacking in the science. What don't we know about Black and Brown bodies? What don't we know about trans bodies? I need to be honest with my patients about this. For example, some of our standard tests for things like vitamin D deficiency or how we screen people's breasts and chests for cancer are racially biased in ways that harm Black people.

My job as a provider is to look at the evidence that informs my practice and notice where it's absent or incomplete. Health care providers sometimes tend to think of people's health as if it exists in a vacuum; it's my job to find and understand the bigger context for the science I use in my work. When I come to clinic, I need to show up understanding the science and also the lack of science I have about the bodies in front of me. I need to be willing to look things up, to be wrong, to be corrected, and to not feel like I need to be thanked because I am correctable.

Zena: What kinds of choices have you made about working inside and outside of existing systems (e.g., working in a hospital vs. working in a grassroots community-led clinic)? What has this taught you about understanding and meeting the health needs of communities who experience systemic oppression?

Ronica: I think a lot of people get into health care because they know it's a secure job that will allow them to support their families and have relatively stable lives. That's definitely a part of why I got into it, but I also very much reject the idea that I cannot do things outside the system or only choose the most stabilizing ways to practise my trade. That means I'm going to go to protests. I'm going to risk professional sanctions or other consequences by starting health care projects in countries where I'm not licensed when the communities I work with have identified a need. I'm going to provide health care to support community autonomy. I'm going to put myself on the line.

My perspective is that we should not be working a "helping job" only as a way to shield ourselves from the poverty, exclusion, and harm our patients experience. We should be willing to interrupt and end the harm, too.

I believe in being in the line of danger when it comes to doing work that supports communities I believe in and want to work with, and who want to work with me. I know this might sound kind of adventure seeking or something, but what I really mean is, what if the biggest barrier to my patients getting health care or being healthy is police violence? Then I'm going to work toward things like police and prison abolition, and decriminalizing sex work and drug use. I'm going to use my professional status as a health care provider as a tool in this work, like being the one to deal with the police if they show up in a health care setting so my patients don't have to.

I believe in being part of revolutions in the world. I don't mean "revolution" in an ideological sense. I mean being part of international revolutions, being part of revolutionary movements in India, Athens, and Egypt, offering care in places with refugee crises. Being part of alleviating harm for people in these situations in the hope that it will create more room for people to think about systems and create change in the world. That's what health care is about for me. It's about making as many healthy people as possible in the world who can challenge the systems that create a lack of care in their lives.

It means being unrelenting. It means social justice has to be the first thing I think about, not, "Oh, and then I've got to get a little social justice in here." It means looking at the patient in front of me and asking if this person needs racial and economic justice, or other forms of justice in their life. Can I be part of creating a process toward justice for this person? How can I do this with the very few skills I have?

I believe health care providers should be putting our asses on the line. We should be putting our credibility on the line. It's not worth anything if we don't do this. It doesn't make the world a better place because you charged Medicaid to see a patient and gave them medications. It just doesn't. I think a lot of people in health care think they spend a lot of time helping people and actually, we get paid to help people. And that's fine.

If we're working in a capitalist system, which we are, it's not so bad to be supporting ourselves and our families within that system. It's fine but it's not enough. Many of us in the United States, including me, graduate with hundreds of thousands of student debt and have people who depend on us for financial support. I know how crushing this debt can be in our lives, but I still believe we can't wait for it to not exist in order to do work that is crucial to the communities most affected by harmful policies that create or exacerbate poverty.

But I also ask myself, can you do the work for free and care just as much about it? I think there are a lot of people who would say no to that question. I think that's the wrong value system. There is the belief that time is money. I don't believe that you can buy my time. My time is absolutely the most valuable thing I have, and I will give it away freely before I allow myself to spend big chunks of my time doing something I don't like for money. My perspective is that radical health care providers should do whatever we can to decrease the gap between our political beliefs and our actions and be in a practice of constantly examining this gap.

This has been a hard decision-making process for me. It doesn't make me wealthy, that's for sure. It definitely means I've worked as a hotel doorman to make ends meet while being a professor at Yale because I couldn't bring myself to work health care jobs I don't feel passionate about. It also means that academia has undervalued my work because I did not choose a traditional path.

And that's alright. I don't love that these are the options I have in front of me but as somebody who didn't come up with a lot of money, I don't see a way to actually be true to my ethics that also gives me a cushion as much of the time as I might like. I'm willing to not have a cushion. That is a hard decision at times, but it's an okay decision for me to allow myself to feel what it's like to struggle in the world and not be so protected by a relatively well-paying job. Particularly if I feel like it advances what I care about, which is achieving racial and economic justice.

Zena: What sustains you in this work? How do you take care of yourself while doing it?

Ronica: What sustains me in this work is being able to see the change in communities as a result of the work of myself and people in the organizations I work with. When I get passionate about something it's not unusual for me to take a step toward it, and that includes doing international work. Why do I care about the communities I care about? Well, it's pretty hard for me not to care about refugees and migrants at the border. My way of contributing to that care is to show up and provide medical care in those communities. It might be a minor thing for many people, but it's what I have.

It sustains me to know that the work I'm doing is representative of what I'm capable of. I bring the best I can to doing this work. And honestly, it's very gratifying. It feels good to do work I think is important because it fits my value system. So many people are robbed of their autonomy in the world. If I can be part of the process of helping someone have greater access to self-determination and autonomy, I find that very invigorating and sustaining.

Zena: What are your wildest dreams for the health of LGBTQ+ people and communities?

Ronica: My wildest dreams are that people get to have the relationships they want, the sex they want (if they're people who want sex), the enjoyment they want, and the ability to be important in the world as much as they want. People get to lead their lives without having to be worried about consequences because of who they are. And, you know, as soon as I say that, I feel like some people might picture a bunch of white angsty teenagers in North America, but I'm talking about Black, Brown, disabled, purses-falling-from-mouths and built-in-strap-ons queers, or hiding-it-for-their-lives queers all over the world.

People all over the world are dying because of who they are, where they were born, and because they live in contexts that devalue their lives. There are people fleeing all over the world or stuck in one place because of the consequences of capitalism. My wildest dream is that nobody ever has to do this again. I want to live in a world where no person is seen as illegal, there are no borders, no police, and no prisons. I want every person to be safe wherever they are, safe enough that they want to create safety for other people as well, and able to move freely if that's their desire. I want people to feel safe enough to love who they love—friends, family, lovers—and able to intervene when they see an injustice, big or small.

Dreaming Bigger

Body Liberation and Weight Inclusivity in Health Care

Sand C. Chang

I. THE VISION

Imagine this: You schedule an appointment to go to the doctor for a routine exam. You have no anxiety about going because you know the doctor will not make assumptions about your health based on your appearance or body weight. In fact, they won't even be interested in weighing you because they know this is a subpar way to make determinations about your health. Instead, they *listen to you*. They are more interested in what you have to say than the size or shape of your body.

Health care providers universally agree that body mass index (BMI) is an antiquated medical concept not useful or relevant for assessing health. Your providers treat you with respect not despite your body size, but because they work from the understanding that all bodies are worthy. When something is not working well with your body, they prescribe treatments that support your overall health and wellness regardless of the size of your body. Doctors say "I don't know" rather than suggest weight loss as a universal treatment for anything that they don't understand. They have done their own personal work to understand and uproot their own internalized fatphobia because they know they are a part of systems that can perpetuate harm toward patients and understand that systemic transformation starts with each individual.

Concepts like Health at Every Size® (HAES)—a movement based on size and fat acceptance—and weight inclusivity/neutrality are core aspects of the curriculum for anyone training to be a health care provider. It's easy to find a care provider who is fat positive and weight inclusive.

Medical buildings and facilities are inclusive of and welcoming to all body sizes. There are accessible, comfortable chairs in waiting rooms and exam rooms. When you need a particular medical service or surgery, there is equipment strong enough to support bodies at every size. Throughout your entire visit, you trust that the doctors, support staff, and medical and insurance systems care about your emotional and psychological safety. They want you to *feel* comfortable in and connected to your body rather than superficially wanting you to *look* "healthy" to the external world. And you are never, ever asked to step on a scale unless there is a valid clinically indicated reason for doing so.

If you're struggling with food or your body size, shape, or weight, there are resources for you. There are places you can be referred to where you know the providers and staff are all affirming of not only queer and trans people, but also BIPOC, disabled, and neurodivergent people and people who are some or all of the above. And these identities are reflected in the provider teams themselves.

Harm reduction is the larger framework that guides treatment discussions and decisions. The aim of the care you receive is not to fix you or make you conform in any way, but to help reduce and remove barriers to resilience and embodiment, and to foster your capacity to trust your body. Everyone can easily access care whenever they need it, no matter what their income is or where they live.

You feel like a person, not a diagnosis, a number, or a problem. The health care professionals you work with ask you to be a collaborative partner with your lived experience being valued just as much as, if not more than, anything they learned from a textbook. You are not blamed in any way for your suffering. You feel comfortable speaking honestly with your providers about what you are feeling and experiencing because you trust that they are committed to understanding and helping you.

What I've invited you to imagine with me is not our current reality. There's much to be desired when it comes to the ways our health and medical systems are able to serve queer and trans people regarding body size, shape, and weight. Most people—including many health care providers—are largely unconscious when it comes to calling out diet culture as a problem or even recognizing it as a product of white supremacy and colonialism. To move toward a world in which weight stigma does not permeate our experiences of seeking medical care, we need to wake up to the ways in which we have all been affected by diet culture and fatphobia and actively participate in creating systems that honour our queer and trans bodies at any and all sizes.

II. MY STORY

I was only five when Dr Small, my pediatrician, informed my mom that I needed to lose weight. With his white-man, white-coat authority, he stated this as a fact. I don't remember exactly how I felt sitting there hearing Dr Small appraise my small round body, but I remember that I didn't like him. Even at that young age, I knew that he was communicating bad news. It would never dawn on me or my immigrant mother to question the validity of this proclamation coming from a white man in authority, and a medical doctor at that.

My first attempts to lose weight started soon after, as my older sister had picked up a calorie-counting book around that time and I thought I should join her. I can still picture the thick, red-and-white paperback book with charts and tables for every food item imaginable and worn, dog-eared pages that soon became my bible. As hard as I tried to count my calories and stick to it, I would inevitably "break" my diet, leading me to think that I was the problem. *If only I had more willpower. If only I didn't love food so much. If only I could follow the rules, I wouldn't fail. Maybe I just needed to try harder.*

I could just stop here, as the story repeated itself throughout my life for years, with a few variations. Add in some food restriction, reducing food to "points," a lot of compulsive exercise, but the result was the same: lose weight, get showered with praise, regain more weight than I'd lost, be confronted with silence from others, feel a sense of failure. Rinse and repeat.

This is how diet culture works.

My story is not unique, but I didn't know that then. I didn't know that my efforts to control my food and weight were responses to the deeply internalized message that my body was the biggest problem in my life. I didn't know that the more I trusted in the latest diet or nutrition trends, the less I trusted in my body. And I didn't know that my "failures" had little to do with my inherent individual weakness and more to do with the colonialism, white supremacy, mind-body dualism/subjugation, ableism, capitalism, and fatphobia that produce and reproduce diet culture.

My ability to recognize both the extent to which diet culture had affected me and the need to seek help was complicated by a number of external factors. First off, fatphobia is so rampant and normalized in East Asian cultures that I felt I deserved it when my extended family scrutinized, ridiculed, and even pinched (ouch!) my body fat. However, the barriers to accessing care are greater for so many other people who do not have the advantages that class and educational privilege, relative-thin privilege, and the proximity to whiteness that being a lighter-skinned person of colour living in an average-size body have afforded me.

Even the so-called eating disorder "recovery" field that I discovered in my early twenties became a barrier to me seeing the ways in which my healing from my eating disorder was still steeped in fatphobia. It allowed me to take on the narrative of having a food and exercise addiction and that weight loss and a restrictive food plan would keep me in line. Even though I was no longer exercising excessively through the many injuries I sustained, I was still preoccupied with chasing a "normal" weight. I even became an eating disorders therapist, thinking I could draw on my own experiences to help others with officially diagnosable eating disorders, completely unaware that I was engulfed in healthism and internalized fatphobia. My own biases were barriers to helping others find true food and body liberation. Now I understand that I was one among many eating disorder professionals who have unrecognized, untreated eating disorders of their own due to the medical and mental health field's very limited conception of what constitutes a problem.[188]

III. RECOGNIZING DIET CULTURE AND REDEFINING DISORDERED EATING

Diet culture is so pervasive that we don't even know we are living in it. It makes each one of us a promise: *if you lose weight, you will be healthy.* It brainwashes us into believing that there is nothing so virtuous as being thin and that health guarantees happiness. It then follows that if we can only take control of our food and our bodies, we will be safe from the many systems of oppression that tell us that our bodies aren't worthy or good enough.

Healthism, sizeism, fatphobia, weight bias—whatever you want to call it—did not start with the grapefruit diet, or Twiggy, or Atkins, or Richard Simmons. In *Fearing the Black Body: The Racial Origins of Fat Phobia* (2019), Sabrina Strings makes the case that fatphobia was used as a tool of social control during the Enlightenment era. Body size and shape was used as a way to differentiate white women and Black women, based on the racist myth that Black bodies were inferior or savage, thereby justifying their enslavement.

The policing of food and bodies is also rooted in the colonization of Indigenous people and the erasure of their food traditions. The foods and eating customs of Indigenous cultures were deemed "dirty" and were to be "cleaned up" by colonizers. For example, Christopher Columbus feared that European settlers in North America would become more like Indigenous people if they kept eating Indigenous food.[189] It's not difficult to connect this to our culture's current euphemism for dieting: "clean" eating. What's even more insulting is that the wellness industry has appropriated some of the very traditions and practices of Indigenous communities that colonizers disparaged or even prohibited, all with the promise of—you guessed it—weight loss. It's not just the big diet industry, however; some grassroots food activism is also laden with healthist and fatphobia messaging, claiming that obesity is a problem that did not exist prior to colonialism.

The ideals and behaviours promoted by diet culture are inaccessible to most of us. Everything comes at a cost: organic food, cleanses, the newest exercise craze. The assumption is that we are all cis, white, straight, able-bodied people with time and money to spend striving to meet impossible standards. Or that we are all aspiring to look like people with these dominant culture identities and that our own self-hatred just might be the fuel we need to conform to these impossible standards. Most of the fatphobic so-called "solutions" to being at a larger weight rest on the assumption that the individual is to blame for their problems and that they hold the sole responsibility of fixing themselves.

Diet culture has gotten sneakier over time, telling us that "self-love" and "self-care" are the ways to take care of our bodies (without explicitly naming that we should be ashamed of our bodies or our habits as they presently are). The so-called "body positivity" or "BoPo" movement has even co-opted fat activism while divesting it of its history and roots in political activism. The diet industry does not want us to know that 77 to 95 percent of intentional weight loss efforts are not only unsuccessful in the longer term, but often cause even more weight gain, medical problems, and harm to mental health.[190]

One of the most palpable and unfortunately all-too-common examples of how diet culture harms queer communities is the way in which archaic (and racist) BMI and weight requirements[191] are used to systematically deny life-affirming and life-saving surgeries for trans and nonbinary people in larger/fat bodies despite no empirical basis for this practice.[192] This is all done, of course, under the guise of health or safety: that is, "protecting" people from their dangerously fat bodies. Though the BMI was never designed to be an indicator of how individuals' bodies function, it is often used uncritically as a standard by which bodies are deemed healthy or unhealthy.

Despite the commonly held myth that eating disorders only affect cis, white, straight, middle- to upper-middle-class abled women, in reality eating disorders affect people of all cultures, classes, ages, genders, and dis/abilities. People who are typically undiagnosed or underdiagnosed are those who don't fit the eating disorder stereotype; this includes trans, queer, BIPOC, poor people, and cis men. And let's not forget that fat people (people who the medical industry deem as *needing* to lose weight) are often *encouraged* to develop disordered eating habits. When people in larger bodies do report symptoms of disordered eating, they are frequently neither believed nor given any viable treatment options.

Eating disorders are typically diagnosed using criteria so stringent and culturally biased that most people with disordered eating, even those who fit the eating disorder stereotype, aren't recognized as having a problem. Anyone who doesn't fit the strict criteria of anorexia nervosa, bulimia nervosa, or binge eating disorder typically falls through the cracks and does not get the support or attention they need. This sometimes leads to double standards in treatment. Take, for example, a thin person and a fat person who exhibit the exact same restrictive food behaviours. The thin person, especially if they dip below 85 percent of a supposed "normal" body weight, would likely be recognized as having anorexia and treatment would encourage them to eat to restore weight, whereas the fat person would be praised and encouraged to keep restricting.

The assessment of eating disorders (by researchers and clinicians) is also overly individualistic. Medical and mental health providers blame the individual for their pathology, their "distorted" body image, or their "compulsive" behaviours. It can be a stretch for providers to even name that expectations for how bodies are supposed to look are based on extremely unrealistic standards perpetuated by the media. Even with this admission, it is still the individual's *internalization* of these ideals that is seen as sick or disordered. The concept of "body image" is extremely limiting, only focusing on one's self-perception and denying the significance of the social contexts and experiences of marginalization that create an environment of toxic shame. We cannot simply change our "body image" if the world continues to shame us for having our (fat, BIPOC, queer, trans, disabled, etc.) bodies in the first place.

Queer and/or BIPOC activist or radical communities are not immune to internalizations of fatphobia or the development of eating disorders. Minority stress has been shown to be associated with binge eating in lesbian and bisexual women.[193] It has also been associated with cisgender gay men's body-image concerns (i.e., pressures to have a lean and muscular body) related to portraying a particular kind of masculinity.[194] Trans men within LGBTQ+ communities may experience a similar kind of minority stress if they feel pressure to express their masculinity in ways that cis gay men do. While many people in trans communities have celebrated a white trans man bodybuilder being on the cover of GQ magazine, this has also had the effect of communicating to other transmasculine people that they, too, need to have chiselled and muscular bodies.

Trans "before and after" photos often boast of success because of the approximation of a cis white beauty ideal. The small but growing body of research we have on eating disorders in trans communities suggests that because of transphobia trans people are at a much higher risk (possibly eight times higher) of having an eating disorder than cis people are. In one large survey, almost 16 percent of transgender participants reported being diagnosed with an eating disorder within the last year, compared to 1.85 percent of cisgender heterosexual women and 0.55 percent of cisgender heterosexual men.[195]

In a world that constantly shames us for our bodies, genders, or sexualities, we can trick ourselves into thinking that we are "taking control" and that achieving a certain body ideal is liberation. It is far from that.

For those of us who face multiple forms of oppression, developing eating disorders is not simply wanting our bodies to meet the impossible aesthetic ideal associated with people in dominant culture. Queer and trans people don't develop disordered eating simply because we want to assimilate to cisgender, heteronormative culture. Of course, appearances can be and often are part of the picture. But when we attribute eating disorders solely to the desire for our bodies to look a certain way, the conversation stops. And we miss out on opportunities for crucial conversations about the connections between eating disorders, trauma, and survival.

IV. EATING DISORDERS AS SURVIVAL

Eating disorders help us to survive trauma and oppression. For queer and trans folks, the way we both conceptualize and heal from eating disorders must account for the ways we are harmed by systems of power.

Eating disorders help us to cope with everyday microaggressions and macroaggressions. They help us to get by in the face of food insecurity. They can keep us safe in a world in which being read as queer or trans can mean life or death. For many people, disordered eating or behaviours are attempts at shape control, which are attempts to blend in and not become a target.

For many of us, eating disorder "treatment" that aims to strip us of the very armour that has allowed us to stay alive, can actually cause more harm if there isn't an adequate substitute or systemic change to help us to safely exist in the world. Treatment cannot simply be aimed at challenging our "distorted thoughts" or symptom reduction or cheerleading body positivity. Treatment approaches that aim at skills training (e.g., dialectical behaviour therapy) and challenging unhelpful thought patterns that fuel an eating disorder (e.g., cognitive behavioural therapy) are often crucial, but they are not enough for a true sense of feeling safe and at home in one's body.

Most mainstream treatment approaches perpetuate white supremacist, capitalist systems of harm. Fat people are told that they are holding on to their fat as protection and that if they worked through their trauma, the weight would fall away. Thin people are told they need to restore their weight but they are not to go beyond an established "upper limit." When we demonize "emotional eating," there is an inherent assumption that the individual can get to a calm, neutral state at all times when their body needs or wants to be fed. Sometimes "emotional eating" is harm reduction.

Our disorders and symptoms, the things that we feel shame about, were once what helped us to get through the night. We might still be in survival mode. Or, we might have a hard time recognizing that we no longer need to be in survival mode. But before we move on, we might have to pay respect and allow ourselves to grieve how we have been called to protect ourselves in ways that are simultaneously brilliant and destructive.

V. FINDING OUR WAY OUT

There is a beautifully growing movement of liberation-centred approaches to dismantling diet culture and fatphobia. We might hear the words body positivity/acceptance, Intuitive Eating (IE), Health at Every Size® (HAES), Body Trust®, weight neutrality/inclusivity, and the list goes on. These approaches all aim to create a world in which people in larger bodies are afforded the same respect and privileges granted to people in smaller bodies. However, these approaches and philosophies vary greatly in terms of truly addressing fatphobia's white supremacist and colonial roots. They are still, for the most part, centred on straight white cis women to the exclusion of BIPOC and queer and trans people.

How do we get to a place of body liberation for all? How can we make a weight-inclusive, fat-positive health care experience a shared reality?

We cannot try to reform current systems to make them "nice" or "inclusive" to people who aren't straight, cis, or white. We need a complete overhaul and a new system that centres the needs of those who have been most impacted by white supremacy, colonialism, and fatphobia. We cannot simply aim to train providers to do better today; we must look at education systems, research methods and funding, and resource redistribution. We must all look at the ways in which we are complicit in perpetuating diet culture and body shame. We need to be committed to dismantling the problem from all angles and creating something new and different, something that goes beyond the vision I have offered you at the beginning of this piece. I offer the following action steps only as a beginning because visioning work must be a collective process. I hope that you will take what you've read here to inspire your own movements, to start conversations with people in your lives or the systems in which you work, to dream bigger together, to do better together.

ACTIONS FOR PROVIDERS

Action steps for providers who are committed to actively dismantling diet culture within themselves and in their patient communities:

1. Engage your curiosity. Get suspicious about everything you've ever been taught about weight or fatness. Understand that becoming a true advocate and accomplice requires a great deal of unlearning of what may be viewed as "truths" by many leaders in the medical and health fields. This includes challenging what has been viewed as the truth by science, as scientific evidence and perspectives are not neutral but rather situated within societal structures and systems of oppression.

2. Read as much as you can about body liberation and nondominant approaches to thinking and talking about weight in medicine. Familiarize yourself with Health at Every Size® and Intuitive Eating.

3. Consciously check yourself and interrogate when you make assumptions about a person's health based on their appearance, weight, or BMI.

4. Go beyond "body image" and look at the ways in which your relationship to your own food and body are situated in white supremacy and colonialism. Read books by BIPOC such as *Fearing the Black Body* by Sabrina Strings.

5. Make sure your environments are inclusive for people in larger bodies. This includes waiting rooms, exam rooms, and medical equipment.

6. Unfollow toxic diet culture social media accounts or any media that increases your body shame or body judgment of others. Follow accounts that focus on intersectional body liberation, especially BIPOC accounts.

7. Consciously reallocate your resources (time, money, energy). How can you invest in yourself or your communities and divest from diet culture?

8. Advocate for weight-neutral and inclusive medical training, whether it is medical school curriculum or representation at academic/professional conferences. Consider including weight-neutral texts such as *The Body Is Not an Apology* by Sonya Renee Taylor, *Anti-Diet* by Christy Harrison, or *Sick Enough: A Guide to the Medical Complications of Eating Disorders* by Jennifer Gaudiani in syllabi.

9. Before making any referrals to other providers or organizations, be sure to do labour ahead of time to gauge the extent to which these providers utilize a weight-neutral, fat-positive approach. Set up conversations and ask direct questions. Although there can never be guarantees, it is the responsibility of the provider to try to know as much as possible before offering referrals. When in doubt or if a provider is found to be aligned with an approach that is not fat-affirming, for example, this information can also be provided to patients so that they can make a decision based on informed consent as to whether or not to engage with those providers.

10. Be prepared to need support in pushing back against harmful systems and practices. Find an accountability partner or group to support your body liberation work. Come up with concrete goals and schedule times to discuss triumphs and challenges on a regular basis.

RECOGNIZING DIET CULTURE AND INTERNALIZED FATPHOBIA: QUESTIONS TO ASK YOURSELF

These questions are meant to call attention to the insidious ways that our societies are steeped in diet culture and fatphobic ideals. If you answer "yes" to any of these questions, you may want to more closely examine your relationship to food and bodies.

Value judgments

- Do I categorize foods as "good" or "bad"?
- Do I believe that people are morally obligated to be in good health?

Reinforcing diet culture as the norm

- Do I say things like, "Oh, just start again tomorrow" or "It's okay to cheat!"?
- Do I tell people they "deserve" to eat certain food?

Fatphobia or internalized weight stigma

- Do I categorize bodies as "healthy" based on weight?
- Do I use slurs like "obese" or "morbidly obese" without a critical lens of how this pathologizes fatness?
- Do I feel uncomfortable with the idea of gaining weight? Of being fat?

Enacting more subtle forms of diet culture

- Do I promote "clean eating" or "fitness" or a "lifestyle change" with weight loss as a desired outcome?
- Do I promote cutting out whole food groups?

Revolution through Health Care

Interview with Anita "Durt" O'Shea, St. James Infirmary

Anita O'Shea is deputy director of St. James Infirmary (SJI), a peer-based nonprofit organization that serves sex workers throughout the San Francisco Bay Area. SJI is the first occupational health and safety clinic in the United States run by sex workers for sex workers. Our conversation offers an exciting vision for what sex worker–led health care grounded in a commitment to social justice and harm reduction can look like.

Zena: Tell me the story of how St. James Infirmary came to be. How was the leadership of sex workers integral to its formation?

Anita: Sex worker activists like Margo St. James, Priscilla Alexander, and Gail Pheterson first came up with the idea of a sex worker–run clinic in the mid-1980s. Several years later, a sex worker was arrested and forcibly tested for sexually transmitted infections (STIs) in jail without her consent and without being given a reason for a blood draw. This sparked the creation of a more compassionate and harm reduction–based way of providing health care to sex workers, driven by the sex worker movement and passionate health care activists.

Because one individual sex worker spoke up and reached out to COYOTE (Call Off Your Old Tired Ethics), a local sex workers' rights organization, the entire sex worker community was able to benefit.

This peer-based model was hard won, but with support from the city's department of public health, the project has continued for over twenty years since our clinic first opened in 1999.

Zena: What kinds of programs and services can people access at SJI? How are they different from what you might find at a conventional health clinic? How does your approach help meet the health needs of queer and trans sex workers?

Anita: We offer a wide range of programs: primary health care, transgender health care including access to hormones, mental health services (talk therapy and groups), HIV testing and linkage to care, STI testing and treatment, acupuncture and massage, syringe access and harm-reduction supply distribution, housing for trans and gender nonconforming people, and outreach and community engagement.

Participants can access our services at the same time. For example, someone could come to our drop-in space, have a hot meal, and take home groceries, clothing, and condoms, while also having the opportunity to get a checkup from a clinician, acupuncture treatments, or just talk with one of our peer counsellors.

Our services are driven by what sex workers see as most needed. For example, the group Mujeres Latinas En Acción was entirely conceived of by Latinx sex workers to provide a space for TransLatinas to gather, eat, be in community, and build leadership and empowerment among each other. The Our Trans Home project houses transgender and gender nonconforming and nonbinary people. It is spearheaded by current and former sex workers to provide one of the most necessary and sought-after services in our city to the most underserved population: housing for trans people.

SJI also holds workshops for sex workers, but some of our most important work is community engagement to help educate health care workers, students, artists, and corporate groups about the importance of sex worker rights and the fights for harm reduction and against criminalization. The San Francisco Bay Bad Date List was a sex worker–led project, again with the support of the city of San Francisco via the Department on the Status of Women. This is a free resource for the community and is extremely necessary when the police refuse to hear sex workers' reports of violence and violation. The sex worker community has historically had to depend on itself to meet its needs and protect itself.

The Outreach team at SJI provides essential services to sex workers on the streets of San Francisco (on the "stroll") because we understand the barriers and isolation sex workers experience. As a peer-based community of staff and volunteers, we understand the need to go to where the sex workers are and not wait for them to come to us. It is a slow process of building trust among the community, even as current and former sex workers, because so much trauma and damage has been done to keep us apart.

The main difference between SJI and other more conventional health clinics is that the staff and volunteers often openly identify as sex workers. This allows for more trust, compassion, and understanding to flow between "patients" and "providers." Having staff and volunteers from the trans and queer sex worker community makes our clinic more approachable and enables word-of-mouth outreach within the community.

Zena: SJI's mission is "to meet the needs of people engaged in the sex trade through advocacy, direct services, and social justice." How does that mission—in particular, your commitment to social justice—inform the ways you define what health is and how you provide health care?

Anita: Our mission is based on lived experiences of sex workers and our interactions with health care professionals. We utilize our personal experiences to educate and enact effective and compassionate health care for our participants. We also understand that truly effective and compassionate health care can only happen when our society addresses inequities based on race, gender, sexual identity, age, ability, HIV and immigration status. Without addressing the underlying issues of our society, we will not achieve a true transformation of the health care system.

Zena: Why is decriminalization of sex work an LGBTQ+ health issue?

Anita: Queer and trans people make up a huge population of the sex worker community—75 percent of SJI participants identify as LGBTQ+. Transgender people are harassed and profiled as sex workers by police. The decriminalization of sex work would reduce this level of harassment and stigma against sex workers in general.

Zena: Tell me more about what SJI's peer-based clinic model looks like in practice, and how being peer-based informs how you do your work and helps shift the power imbalances that often characterize health care.

Anita: In practice, being peer-based does not erase inequity or the challenges of any other workplace. There is a lot of stratification within the sex worker community, so sometimes that plays out in a sex worker organization. That being said, SJI attempts to centre the most marginalized of the sex worker community: trans sex workers and sex workers of colour. SJI tries to listen intentionally to our participants and be truly client-centred in our work. As peers, we understand better how to communicate with participants and how information is most effectively shared with them.

Zena: How do the principles of harm reduction inform the way SJI works? What does harm reduction look like in practice at SJI?

Anita: SJI is based in harm reduction because we believe that health care needs to address each individual and not generalize and stereotype an entire community, which often leads to misdiagnosis and alienation between providers and patients. Because we are sex workers, we understand the importance of addressing the needs of our community whether that is to fight for decriminalization of sex work or to provide clean syringes and other safer injection supplies to anyone who needs them (not just sex workers).

The emphasis at SJI is to avoid any kind of judgment of our participants based on sex work or drug use. Being a nonjudgmental space is an ongoing process and not always a guarantee. But any staff or volunteers who start at SJI are given a full training on harm reduction and we emphasize the importance of creating a safer space for sex workers.

Often our participants tell us that SJI is the only place that they feel comfortable to be themselves. This is a huge point of pride in our organization, and we work really hard to maintain this attempt at safer space for sex workers.

Zena: SJI has a stated commitment to the liberation of trans people of colour. How are you putting this commitment into practice? How is it shaping the ways you define health and organize around the health of trans folks of colour?

Anita: This commitment is an ongoing goal and is enacted through hiring staff and recruiting to our board of directors. SJI also focuses on providing care to trans people of colour by going to where they are in the community, in the kinds of groups and events that we host. This is an ongoing process, and we are learning a lot as we go. Recently we decided to formally recruit a consultant to help us with equity training. SJI is also the fiscal sponsor for three organizations that are led by Black trans women: the Trans Activists for Justice and

Accountability (TAJA) Coalition, Transgender Gender-variant and Intersex Justice Project (TGIJP), and the Transgender District.

Zena: What are some of the challenges queer and trans sex workers tend to experience in accessing knowledgeable, respectful, and dignified health care?

Anita: The mainstream health care industry often generalizes about peoples' experiences and discriminates based on gender and sexuality. The challenge of doctors assuming everyone is straight has decreased somewhat, but transphobia in health care still very much needs to be addressed.

Sex workers often keep their profession private from their health care providers for fear of being shamed. I have encountered several participants (clients/patients) at SJI who tell me they have never told a doctor about being a sex worker. Some tell me that when they did talk about their profession, they were told they shouldn't be doing that work. Most recently a participant told me she had been seeing a doctor to help her stay off drugs and when she told him she got a job as a stripper, he told her she shouldn't be working there and to stay away from "people like that."

The conflation of sex work with drugs and violence in our society affects how health care professionals perceive sex workers. These professionals are not usually trained on ideas of harm reduction and meeting people where they're at. The stigma and shame sex workers are subjected to within our society very much extends to the health care sector.

Zena: What advice, tips, or strategies would you offer to queer and trans sex workers on how to advocate for their own health when they're accessing health care?

Anita: I would advise queer and trans sex workers to take notes and be prepared to advocate for yourselves and/or bring an advocate (trusted friend or family member or service provider like a case manager) with you to your appointment. I would also recommend screening your health care providers when possible. Interview them and ask relevant questions like: "Do you have experience working with queer/trans/sex worker patients?" "Have you ever helped someone get on hormones? Or gender-affirming surgery?" Based on their answers you could decide that they may not be the best provider for you. This is especially relevant with therapists. It's important to "shop around" to find the right mental health provider if possible. Sex workers can also call upon organizations like SJI or their local sex worker advocacy group, if there's one in their area, to help them identify providers who are culturally competent in caring for sex workers.

Zena: Health care providers rarely receive information or training about sex work or sex workers (especially information or training that centres sex workers' expertise and knowledge). What advice, tips, or strategies would you offer to health care providers who want to be better allies to the queer and trans sex workers they care for?

Anita: The main tip I have for health care providers is to keep your personal opinions to yourself! You can provide excellent care to someone without them ever knowing that you dislike their choice in hair style; please do the same when it comes to someone's work choices. This seems pretty simplistic, but the reality is that sex workers who need health care often have specific needs that have absolutely nothing to do with their profession.

Something I have also learned is that sometimes you may not be the best person to provide health care to a person. For example, if you are a therapist and have many personal biases against sex workers, then you should not be providing care to a sex worker. Even if you are working to unlearn the stereotypes about sex workers, you are probably not the best fit and should be honest with clients and potential clients and make a referral to someone who will be able to work better with the individual.

The main thing to keep in mind: sex workers are just like everyone else! They need medical care just like anyone else and if you suspect any issues like abuse or STIS, you should ask the same questions you would ask anyone else to determine how best to serve the individual. Questions about sex work and sex in general can be very uncomfortable for participants and providers. It's important to be open, caring, patient, and kind.

Sometimes certain terms or language can be confusing. For example, the word "client" can refer to a program participant or a patient but is also the term that sex workers use to refer to their customers. Another example is that LGBTQ+ people have varied terms to refer to sex and genitalia. Sometimes health care providers may need to be specific in questions regarding sexual history. It's not effective to ask someone "Do you have sex with men or women?" Instead, ask questions like "Do you like to give or receive when you are having sex, or do you do both?"

Try to be specific and nonjudgmental in your tone. Practise asking nongendered questions with everyone and stop yourself from making assumptions about people's genders and sexual activities. For example, just because someone identifies as a lesbian doesn't mean they aren't having sex with cis men. This is especially relevant in the sex worker community because many of us identify as lesbians and/or queer women, but we have sex with cis men for money.

Zena: SJI believes in "revolution through health care." What does that revolution look and feel like to you? What are your wildest dreams for the health and health care of queer and trans sex workers?

Anita: The revolution means to me: sex workers in full control of their health care, housing, and safety. Sex workers often have to rely on themselves and community anyways. I think the health care industry could learn so much from sex workers about what true health care means. It means the rights and safety of each individual are guaranteed. Each person has what they need to survive *and* thrive: housing, food, child care, education, health care, community, and joyful activities.

Do You Feel Empowered by Your Job? And Other Questions Therapists Ask Sex Workers

Kai Cheng Thom

"Was it the good kind of sex work, though? Did you feel empowered?" This was the first thing that my white, middle-class lesbian psychotherapist colleague said when I told her I'd done sex work at various times in my life. The question gave me pause: *Was* my sex work experience a good one? *Did* I feel empowered? As a sex worker? As a psychotherapist? Existentially? In the greater scheme of broader society?

And if my answer was "no," might my colleague consider that the fault of my participation in the sex industry, or see it as an intrapsychic failing, the result of developmental trauma?

My former colleague is a strong mental health clinician who is capable of integrating complex understanding of sex work, oppression, and anticapitalism into her work and world view. Yet I believe the anecdote above illustrates the ways that popular and mental health discourse—even (or perhaps, especially) when inflected by queer, anti-oppressive, and other critical lenses—continue to understand sex work and sex workers as a "special" population whose possession of personal agency is more tenuous than the general population's and therefore must remain constantly in question.

This is not to say that those engaged in the sex industry are never denied autonomy in the course of their work—sex workers acknowledge that violence, coercion, and exploitation do occur within their field, as feminist scholar Ann Russo documents in *Feminist Accountability: Disrupting Violence and Transforming Power*.[196] I can recall many moments in my sex work experience where I felt pressured into doing things I wasn't comfortable with (I will note that I can say the same about literally any job I've had), and certainly I've known sex workers who experienced serious violence and trauma while at work.

However, as Russo points out, the responses of service providers, law enforcement, and academics have more often than not contributed to the disempowerment and marginalization of women—and, I would add, people of all genders—who have engaged in labour activities that are commonly considered sex work.

At the heart of this paradigm is the notion that sex work is fundamentally separate from the larger corpus of capitalized labour in general. Perhaps because of its intrinsic association with the erotic (itself always a highly contested category), sex work is considered inherently dangerous and uniquely degrading, an erotophobic (sex-negative) dynamic I'll examine in more detail later on. Sex workers' relationship to their erotic labour is seen as uniquely fraught, with their ability to consent, make choices, and identify their own best outcomes nebulous at best.

This framing of sex work and sex workers results in a wide variety of repercussions in the institutional and interpersonal treatment of sex workers in mental health care and social services. Psychotherapy, counselling, and clinical social work and related professions/ activities are particularly implicated given their contributions to the public and professional understandings of trauma, sexual norms, and capacity for informed consent in relation to sex workers. Furthermore, the "helping professions" play a central role in carrying out projects related to the criminalization and stigmatization of sex work—for example, by providing court-mandated therapy to those convicted of the crime of prostitution (in jurisdictions where providing sexual services is illegal) and by participating in the design and delivery of "exit programs," in policy-making in shelters and other services that may have the cessation of sex work as a criteria for entry, and in the apprehension of children from parents who are sex workers.

In this essay, I outline some important considerations for mental health and social service providers who work or intend to work with individuals engaged or formerly engaged in sex work, as well as for advocates intending to change the sociolegal conditions surrounding the sex industry. Most importantly, service providers will be prompted to consider their own assumptions and positionality in relation to the sex work in a way that strives to move beyond the framework of "cultural competency." Rather than attempting to simply become "friendlier" to sex workers, service providers might consider the ways in which their own labour, and the work of care in general, is closely interrelated with sex work, giving way to potential for mutual learning and solidarity in struggle.

To the professional "helpers"—social workers, counsellors, psychotherapists, and so on—reading this, "solidarity in struggle" might be a familiar phrase if you consider yourself an anti-oppressive practitioner. After all, hasn't anti-oppressive practice recently become a core professional value of contemporary social work, and a growing area of discussion in other mental health and helping disciplines?

If you are an anti-oppressive practitioner, then you likely know this famous quote from Lilla Watson and the Queensland Aboriginal activists group: "If you have come here to help me, you are wasting your time. But if you have come because your liberation is bound up with mine, then let us work together." I've had more than a few managers and supervisors who kept that quote on posters above their desks. But, dear professional helper, I want to ask you: What stakes do social workers and psychotherapists have in "the struggle," exactly? Not only as individuals, but as a class of specialized labourers? What do mental health and social service providers have in common with sex workers?

Little, if any, intradisciplinary literature exists to answer this question, perhaps unsurprisingly, given the amount of social stigma still attached to sexual labour within psychotherapeutic circles. Indeed, the field of mental health and social service provision has become increasingly whorephobic over time, with some professional schools and associations recently making explicit prohibitions against the entry of sex workers to their ranks, as reported by Sophie K Rosa in a 2019 article for *VICE* magazine titled "Sex Workers Make Great Therapists—but They're Locked Out of the Job."[197] These restrictions, made ostensibly for ethical reasons, imply a moral judgment against sex workers, where the "respectable" professions of therapy and social work are raised above the "immoral" professions of erotic labour. It will come as no surprise to mental health providers, then, that I kept my own sex work experience a secret for many years among my colleagues, even while I worked openly as a queer, transgender woman. Some kinds of diversity are more palatable than others.

However, despite such repudiations, the similarities between sex work and social work/psychotherapy are largely self-evident: Social workers, therapists, and sex workers all provide services involving physical and emotional presence, emotional labour, and intimacy to their clients. Some mental health and social service providers may be surprised to learn that many sex workers, furthermore, consider themselves erotic healers and/or educators; and some have even created extensive training programs, written works, and ethical codes, as British psychologist Philip Cox and an anonymous coauthor going by "Aella" point out in their paper "Whore Phobia: The Experiences of a Dual-Training Sex Worker–Psychotherapist."[198] Even intraprofessional shorthand is similar—I enjoy a private laugh whenever I'm reminded that social workers and sex workers both frequently refer to themselves by the acronym "sws" or "swers" in writing, and that sex workers and mental health professionals are often simply termed "service providers" by their clientele.

The parallels run deeper still: Social service providers, mental health clinicians, and sex workers all comprise highly feminized labour forces (though individuals of other genders *do* participate) that are also highly stratified by race, class, education, and other demographic markers. For example, the hypothetical racialized social service worker who staffs overnight shifts at a women's shelter is likely to be paid a fraction of the salary commanded by a doctoral degree–holding psychotherapist in private practice, while also being exposed to vastly higher levels of workplace danger, exploitation by employers, and burnout. Similarly, the "low track" migrant street sex worker is likely to be outearned by a "high class" call girl whose online advertisements display a strong command of upper-middle-class aesthetics.

Street sex workers and other working-class sex workers are also significantly more likely to experience exploitation from managers ("pimps") or clients. However, as Butterfly: Asian and Migrant Sex Workers Support Network observes in its 2018 study of migrant sex workers in Toronto, the majority of sex workers report that most of the abuse they experience comes not from the people they work for or with, but from law enforcement officers.[199] The sex workers surveyed in this study describe being forced to submit to strip searches, physical intimidation, and sexual harassment and assault by police, all in the name of their "safety" and "ending exploitation."

I want to spend a moment reflecting on exploitation: I've been eyed for social work since I was in my mid-teens. A racialized, mentally ill, gender queer youth, I was also remarkably articulate, psychologically precocious, eager to help and to please. The adult service providers whose orbit I floated in were quick to notice and take a shine to me—I was one of those once-in-a-blue-moon clients, the kind it feels both easy and rewarding to work with because I was so traumatized yet seemed to "improve" so quickly. The adults I trusted always seemed to want me in their empowerment initiatives, they were eager to put me on youth councils and committees, they gave me leadership roles despite the fact that I was in way over my head. I was brilliant and gifted, they said. I had so much to offer, they said. Helping was what I was made for.

I came to identify my worth with helping, my lovableness with how much I was able to give and please. It didn't matter that most of my early jobs and roles involved some significant risks—for example, facilitating antihomophobia workshops in high schools as a high school student myself might have required a rather enormous amount of self-disclosure and vulnerability to strangers, but it was all for the cause, wasn't it? And how proud my youth workers were whenever I came back from another successful outing. And if the honorariums they paid me were less than minimum wage, well, it was more money than I'd ever made before, wasn't it? And how lucky was I to get paid to do something that did so much good for other people?

When I got to college age, I knew it was my purpose in life to help and heal other people. In my darker moments, it sort of seemed like that was all I was good for—and all the trusted adults, the wise youth workers and therapists and psychiatrists who mentored me, said I was gifted. They said I was special. My diversity made me fashionable. So "interesting" and "textured," one psychotherapy supervisor called me. A wealthy white psychologist said I was an "ambassador for my people." (She didn't specify which people.) This was how, at twenty-two years old, I began an internship that involved doing therapy with adults who had survived childhood sexual trauma. Although I had no real clinical training, I held sessions for them at night in the windowless basement of a hospital in Montreal. I learned therapy techniques quickly, from videos on the internet and by practising on the job. People were counting me. I had to help.

Some quick number-crunching tells me that I gave over 4,000 hours of unpaid therapy in order to get to paid work as a clinician. By contrast, the very first sex work gig I got paid me $100 for some nude cuddling and a sloppy hand job that I completed in twenty minutes. I almost never think about that first gig now. I still dream about the stories my clients told me in that first unpaid therapy internship I took at twenty-two. Occasionally, I still cry, wondering how they are now, if I'd done enough to help them.

My social work experience isn't every social worker's experience, so I can't claim to speak for the whole social work community. What I can say is that the people around me saw something useful and beautiful that they liked in me, so they took it and used it and I allowed it to happen because I wanted to feel loved and I didn't think I really had choices. What I can say is that my sex work practice started out rough and frightening, but it blossomed into a decent learning experience and a business that paid me lots of cash up front, usually with no strings attached.

Mental health and social work professionals might consider asking themselves the same question that my former colleague asked me: *Do you feel empowered by your work? Is it the good kind?* Similar questions in this vein that professional helpers often ask sex workers include: *Have you ever been exploited by your boss? Is this kind of work your first choice? Do you make a lot of money? Does that make it worth it? Did childhood trauma lead you to this work? Have you ever experienced trauma while on the job? Do clients ever ask you to do things you don't want to do? Do you ever want to stop doing this? What would you do if you needed to leave?*

The point of this line of inquiry is to galvanize serious reflection on the part of helping professionals regarding the nature of whorephobia and whorephobic attitudes, which are often intertwined with well-meaning intentions. Such good intentions are, more often than not, patronizing and infantilizing because they arise from the expectation that sex workers are inherently psychologically damaged and in need of rescue.

Simultaneously, the glamorized archetype of the "empowered," high-class feminist whore whose work is justified by her access to wealth and free-spirited attitude creates an unhelpful distinction that at once forces sex workers to justify themselves through the rhetoric of "empowerment" and occludes the reality that sex work—like all work—exists on a moving spectrum encompassing an infinite range of experiences of agency, exploitation, autonomy, coercion, satisfaction, and disenfranchisement.

Comparing sex work to therapy and social work through a labour relations lens provides some important insight to the nature of late-stage capitalism: No one really "chooses" to work, though some individuals do have access to a limited range of decision-making about what type of work they do, and at what level of compensation. Yet even the most lucrative, rewarding jobs are inflected by coercion and the potential for abuse. The fact that relatively few workers are able to carve out positions that are well remunerated and emotionally fulfilling is not evidence that the system is equitable as a whole; rather, it is a complex phenomenon created at the intersection of individual ingenuity and systemic privilege.

Some more questions for helping professionals: *What would happen if, instead of centring sex work as a uniquely problematic situation encompassing a binary of "victims" and "empowered" actors, you turned your focus to the acquisition of labour rights for all—including those in our own fields? How might the problems commonly attributed to sex work as an industry shift if women, disabled people, queer and trans people, migrants, and people of colour had guaranteed access to their basic needs and quality education through a thriving social welfare network?*

How would your own experience of your working lives change?

In 2019, the Canadian Association of Social Workers (CASW) released a position paper encouraging the Canadian federal government to, among other actions, decriminalize the buying and selling of sexual services between two consenting adults, permanently fund and expand exit strategies for sex workers wishing to leave the industry, and commit to providing all Canadians with a basic minimum income.[200] When I first read the position paper, I wanted to feel hopeful, but in truth, I mostly felt tired and cynical: the paper represents an encouraging step on the part of the social work profession, but it has yet to be taken up in any way by the government or—based on my own experience of colleagues in the field—by the majority of practising social service providers in the country.

And even this relatively bold position continues to frame sex work as fundamentally separate from the rest of the neoliberal capitalist context of our world, thus de-linking it from other issues and struggles that are essential to an accurate understanding of sexual labour, eroticism as a site of capitalist relations, and gender relations.

Social work and the allied mental health professions have played a key role in defining sex work (or "prostitution") as a "special" problem on moral grounds. Indeed, as Stéphanie Wahab points out in her 2002 paper, "'For Their Own Good?': Sex Work, Social Control and Social Workers, a Historical Perspective," the predecessors of the contemporary social service sector were Charity Organization Society workers, settlement workers, and Evangelicals who first began attempting the moral reform and so-called "protection" of sex workers (and primarily women sex workers) starting in the 1800s.[201] These early helping professionals spanned a gamut of viewpoints on sex workers, viewing them as alternatively deviant "fallen women," victims of male aggression, or the subjects of a phenomenon popularly termed "white slavery" (apparently the fate of women of colour and male sex workers, let alone queer and trans sex workers of colour, was not of much concern to early social workers).

Today, sex work abolitionists seem largely housed within almost identical ideological camps to their historic predecessors, though their rhetoric has expanded somewhat to reflect the growing contemporary concern with racial diversity and feminist consciousness. The nonprofit group AFF3RM, which describes itself as a "transnational feminist organization" denounces prostitution (rejecting the term "sex work") as a "practice of morphing the human body itself into both commodity and factory to satisfy an artificial demand." Here, we can identify the rhetorical partitioning off of sex work as a unique, indeed almost magical, form of oppression because of its supposedly exceptional centring of the body as the site of exchange.

Yet a clear-eyed (and not even particularly sophisticated) review of labour reveals that the body is implicated in all forms of labour. The body is, furthermore, restrained, exploited, commodified, and endangered to various degrees by all forms of labour under capital, some of which may be considered degrading (though this is a matter of perspective) and are certainly dangerous. This was particularly true of the COVID-19 pandemic era, in which agricultural workers and long-term care workers—notably, both are labour pools largely populated by migrants—were at high risk of exposure to deadly disease.

It seems, then, that sex work is not truly set apart by its involvement of the body, nor by its exposure to risk, but by its intersection with the erotic—a moral proposition with roots in Christian, colonial attitudes toward sex.

The existence of male, queer, and transgender sex workers, for example, has long been invisibilized by second-wave feminist attempts at abolition. Yet by appreciating the reality that queer and trans people are more likely than the general population to experience economic discrimination that is linked to erotophobia, we become capable of understanding not only *why* queer and trans people are in fact overrepresented in the sex industry, but *how* queer and trans sex workers might experience the impacts of whorephobia, homophobia, and transphobia as overlapping facets of an overall struggle for survival.

I believe that any discussion of sex work as a labour rights issue must include an acknowledgment of the fact that if sex work is real work, as in labour, then it necessarily produces something of value: namely, sex workers' engagement with the body on an erotic level, the provision of a service that is deeply desired and—I would argue—needed by many people, for many reasons. Sex is an integral part of the human experience, and many, if not most, people experience some level of shame and trauma around their sexuality as a result of colonial attitudes toward sex, many of which have been enforced by the social work and psychotherapeutic professions. In the best of circumstances, sex workers open a counternormative space where clients are able to heal and experience erotic pleasure, sometimes for the first time.

When I opened my sex work practice (yes, it was a *practice* involving the development and application of a high level of professional skill) for the second time, I had the financial resources and social skills to operate from a place of relative safety and control. I sold a unique service that was a combination of exploration for people, mostly men, whose desires fell outside of both normative heterosexuality and normative homosexuality, and sexual trauma healing. My work involved the skilful use of fantasy, loving touch, and intimate discussion—opening a private world that my clients had rarely or never experienced, in which it was both safe and encouraged to find one's own unique erotic expression. It was, in other words, not unlike psychotherapy, except that it touched a place inside people that conventional therapy cannot reach and does not dare to go.

Were there clients who were threatening or pushy? Yes, a few. Then again, as a social worker, I experienced physical violence, harassment, and stalking from some clients. Were there days I did not enjoy my job? Oh, yes. As a social worker, though, there were also days I did not want to work, and the work I did in that role was compensated at the barest fraction of my hourly rate as a sex worker. Is my experience rare among sex workers? Perhaps, though more sex workers (and fewer social workers) find both meaningful work and reasonable working conditions than the general public might think. The point is that my experience in sex work was possible for me as a result of favourable social conditions, which means that it could and ought to be possible for all. The point is that my experience in social work was the result of negative social conditions, which means that helping professionals reading this ought to take a long, hard look at the culture of the field.

It is imperative that mental health and social service providers as a collective acquire a deeper understanding of the mechanisms of whorephobia as a labour rights issue, as well as of the value of sex workers' expertise and contributions to society through their work. Otherwise, we run the risk of becoming trapped in a dualistic model of "good versus bad" sex work that elides the complex and heterogeneous reality of sex workers' actual experiences and perpetuates the "saviour" mentality that infantilizes sex workers and creates dangerous pathways toward denying their capacity for agency and informed consent. We also stand to lose the opportunity to build rich relationships of solidarity with sex-working communities whose resilience and ingenuity might hold the possibility of leading us to better praxis and greater freedom.

As the contemporary era moves toward ever-greater socioeconomic inequality and cries for revolutionary restructuring, the "helping professions" of social work and mental health care are entering a crisis of professional identity—will they remain static, thus acting as handmaidens of the status quo, or will they evolve in the direction of social transformation?

I have some final thoughts for social workers and mental health professionals: *What would happen if you stopped thinking of sex workers as a population in need of rescue, and started thinking of them as colleagues and fellow care workers, siblings in the struggle for a better world? What would it take for you to feel liberated enough to pursue such partnerships in the spirit of equality and authenticity? Is your kind of social work and/or mental health work the "good" kind, the kind you hoped to be doing when you entered the field? Do you feel empowered to make social change? Does your job empower you?*

Borrowed Wisdom

Using Lessons from Queer History and Community in Suicide Intervention

Carly Boyce

I was in grade seven the first time someone told me they wanted to die. My friend, who was bubbly and hilarious, slammed her locker on a Friday afternoon and when I said, "See you Monday," she answered, "Maybe, if I don't kill myself by then."

Three years later it was my turn to be uncertain I could survive my weekends, a struggle I breathed not a single word of while it was most acute. In fact, I did the opposite, creating an elaborate and convincing ruse that I was doing JUST FINE THANK YOU. I have never felt more alone than I did while living inside that fiction. I didn't trust anyone not to flip out, not to tell.

Like many suicidal people, I did not wish to die, precisely; I just couldn't imagine any other way out. I felt like I had no control, no support, and no choices. It took me years to tell anyone else that I had seriously considered ending my life, but it was like other suicidal people could smell it on me. As if by magic, we found each other. I can't count how many friends and community members I have been in this with since.

Twenty years into doing suicide intervention in my communities, and five years into teaching about it, here are six lessons I hope can guide you when supporting someone who is feeling suicidal, whether you're a layperson caring for a friend, or a health care worker supporting LGBTQ+ communities (or anyone in between).

LESSON ONE:
SILENCE = DEATH

Breaking socially enforced silence is a powerful act of resistance and solidarity with folks who are living something unspeakable, and breaking taboos is queer as fuck! AIDS Coalition To Unleash Power (ACT UP) taught us this lesson about HIV in the '80s and I came to it through my poz pals. Speaking aloud the unspeakable breaks the spell of stigma—if only for a moment—and stigma is part of what is killing our communities. People in a supportive role are not alone in our fear of speaking suicide aloud; people who are actively suicidal may also be afraid to say the word, sometimes unable to seek support for fear of triggering others. But I want to tell you this; saying the word "suicide" is not the spell you think it is. It is not an invocation of suicide, but permission to break the pervasive silence around it.

Many suicidal people experience relief at being invited to talk about their suicidality, *even if they don't actually talk to you about it!* The invitation to talk about suicide is itself a powerful intervention that says: someone is willing to listen; someone is not afraid to talk about this; someone cares whether I live or die. We all have the power to break this silence, and talk more openly about suicide with our friends, families, communities, and clients. I encourage everyone to practise talking about suicide, so that when moments arrive when we need to talk about it, the words don't feel quite so clumsy in our mouths.

If you haven't had much practice talking about suicide, I encourage you to find a moment that feels low-stakes to give it a try. You can talk to your hairbrush or your cat. Your recipe is this: an expression of care plus a direct question. Here is an example: "Hey, I care about you a lot, and I know you're dealing with some heavy stuff right now. Are thoughts of suicide coming up for you?" Choose the words that most suit your communication style and your relationship with the person you're talking to.

LESSON TWO:
BINARIES ARE BULLSHIT

I'm not just talking about the gender binary here (though it is extremely bullshit), but about dualistic thinking that we use as a shortcut, instead of working toward nuanced understanding. We do this more when things are escalated and we feel like we don't have time for complexity. Dualistic thinking—thinking in either/or binaries—positions people who are suicidal as fragile, at risk, and needing rescue, while support people are framed as saviours, holding ultimate decision-making power and responsibility. We all know that the Venn diagram of those seeking and giving help has a whole lot of overlap, but we can slide into simplistic thinking when faced with someone we care about struggling with suicidality.

Drug user advocates and consumer-survivors of mental health systems in particular have made it abundantly clear that connecting with people who have shared even a shred of our experiences can bring a sense of deep relief, not necessarily from the suffering itself but from the isolation that magnifies it. Peer support challenges the binary assumption that suicidal people need support from people who are not and never have been suicidal. Suicidal people are actually experts at staying alive in impossible circumstances; they do it every single day. I encourage supporters to resist the urge to take on the responsibility for the survival of someone who tells you they are thinking about suicide, because this approach devalues their skills and their agency. As supporters, we do not need to be in complete control or think of the people we support as helpless. It's not useful, and it's also not true.

How we understand and assess risk in health care settings is another place where false binaries can come into our thinking and cause harm. Health care practitioners are taught a fairly uniform risk assessment strategy and use it to either deny or impose services;

people are seen either as "attention seeking" and not really in need of help, or as in danger, and in need of services whether or not they consent to them. Risk is not a yes/no question, but a deeply complex spectrum, though western medicine offers us either a crisis response or no response at all. Many of us need, and might consent to, something in between.

Notice if you get sucked into binary thinking, as this is more often a sign of your own distress than it is a fair assessment of the person you are supporting. Don't take on the full responsibility for "saving the life" of someone who is suicidal. You do not have to be perfect to be helpful. Be honest about the places you feel challenged. If you are a health care practitioner working with people who are suicidal, think about how to challenge the practices and policies around the care you provide that operate on these binary assumptions.

LESSON THREE:
BODIES ARE WISE

Indigenous cultural producers have taught me about how separation from our bodies, and, by extension, from relationship to the land we live on, is an ongoing violence perpetrated by colonial systems. They taught me that it is the cultures of whiteness and capitalism that demand that we be productivity machines and reinforce the idea that the needs of our bodies are an inconvenience to be minimized. Personally, my entry point into learning about the body as valuable, wise, and connected to the context around it (i.e., the land) came through working with bodyworkers from various lineages (especially acupuncturists), and through my experiences in leatherdyke community. These experiences have taught me about the power and possibility of reconnecting with my own body; that it contains wisdom that can help me make choices, if I can slow down and pay attention to it. Just as relevant in support as in sex, are questions like: Does this feel good? How do I know what good feels like? What would it be like, to treat our bodies more like pets than like pests?

A suicidal urge can be understood as part of the wisdom of the body. In health care settings, we quickly leap to the idea that a suicidal thought is pathological and must be eliminated or cured, and yet we know many people become suicidal as an embodied response to living in circumstances that are intolerable or having traumatic experiences that cannot be digested. It is the suicidal part that tells us—loud and clear—this is not okay; I cannot tolerate this. Our world is full of intolerable circumstances, especially for those most marginalized. What shifts if we think about the suicidal part as being attuned to suffering, or attuned to injustice? This gives us more space as supporters to engage with what hurts, rather than trying to squash the suicidal urge. For me, planning my own death felt like building an escape pod, and knowing this escape pod existed helped me to survive the circumstances I was stuck in until something could change.

In moments of emotional overwhelm, many of us forget, or are otherwise unable, to attend to the needs of our bodies. When our bodies are less resourced (i.e., hungry, tired, cold), it is more difficult to access their wisdom. Someone in a workshop once shared the survival strategy of hugging their dog real close when they feel their worst. It helps them pace their breathing, notice their body, be reminded of connection, and when they feel a little calmer, to eat, drink, and go outside.

When supporting someone in a crisis, I encourage you to check in with body needs. Would the person you are supporting be steadier if they had shelter, nourishment, rest, touch, motion, or stillness? Remember, as a supporter, you, too, have a body, and your body also has needs.

LESSON FOUR:
CONSENT CHANGES EVERYTHING,
AND BOUNDARIES ARE TRUST-BUILDING

I don't just want the consent of suicidal people to matter in our inter-actions of support; I also want support people to know that you, too, are allowed—encouraged even—to know, communicate, and honour your boundaries. My favourite definition of consent comes from somatics practitioner and facilitator Hannah Harris-Sutro, who says it is the intersection of capacity (what we are able to do) and desire (what we want to do).

You cannot do everything, even if you want to. Especially if you live, love, and/or work in marginalized communities. Supporting and serving our communities to thrive is a long game, and we can't burn everyone out. We must grow the team of people who can and will speak openly about suicide so we can collectively hold this suf-fering and hopefully, hopefully, transform it. You must consent to the support you offer, and you must get consent from the people you support about what that looks like. Queer sex radicals have taught me about how much messier and more complicated consent is when people are feeling fucked up, using substances, or otherwise not in their most regulated state. Negotiating in advance is a genius strat-egy we can borrow from BDSM to build advance directives with our close people (more on this in Lesson Five).

The support you can offer when you are operating within your capacity is better than the support you can offer when you are exhausted, overextended, or resentful. Holding your boundaries serves the support work you do, and the relationships you do it in. Also, having and holding sturdy boundaries makes you infinitely more trustworthy as a support person. If you are clear about what you can (and cannot) do, and you follow through, people who are struggling—especially people who worry about burdening others, a common concern for chronically suicidal people—can feel safer reaching out to you because they believe that you won't overcommit and then bail or give support out of a feeling of guilt or obligation and then later resent it.

When supporting suicidal people, ditch questions like "What do you need?" because, though this is earnest and loving, it is also vague and difficult to answer, especially by someone in distress, and most especially by someone who does not feel worthy of care. Instead, ask yourself: Do I have the desire to offer support? What kind? What parts of what I desire do I have capacity for? Then make a few specific, concrete offers. For example: "I can bring you a roast chicken for us to share, we can watch your favourite movie together on FaceTime, or I can sit with you while you call your therapist. Would any of these be helpful?" This provides a kind of boundary that isn't a rejection, but is actually an offer of care.

LESSON FIVE:
POLICE DO NOT PROTECT US

Until 1972, suicide was illegal in Canada, including attempted suicide. The settler state's first attempt at preventing something is to criminalize it, rather than working to change the circumstances that spark it. We see this in drug use, homelessness, and suicide. The creation of criminals from people who are suffering is a violence of colonial and carceral societies. Police are still often called to respond to mental health crises, and too often this results in people in crisis being arrested, or even killed—this is much more likely if the people in distress are Black, Indigenous, poor, or disabled. People marginalized by racism, classism, or ableism are more likely to be viewed as dangerous—rather than in danger—when in distress. My consciousness around abolition has been raised by people I love who have been incarcerated, in the criminal (in)justice system as well as in mental health systems, and by the work of Black liberation movement leaders.

I'm writing this in a political and historical moment when the violence of police forces—most significantly in relation to Black and Indigenous people—is being exposed. And yet, most mainstream suicide intervention programs will tell you to call 911 when you are in over your head. Mandated reporting from health care practitioners is a way that these workers are enlisted as a form of police, to find, report, or incarcerate dangerous people. When people show up at emergency rooms in suicidal crisis, they can be put in seventy-two-hour lockup against their will. A few people I know have found this useful. Many others have found it violent, unsafe, pathologizing of their queerness or gender, and that it blocked access to community support and made them feel powerless and alone.

I encourage folks to make plans in advance with their friends, family members, and communities about who they want to be contacted, and how they want to be treated, in a moment of crisis. Some questions that might be useful are: How will I know if you're not okay? What changes should I watch for in your behaviour or mood? Do you have a doctor or therapist or acupuncturist or herbalist or other kind of healer or health care worker you have a good relationship with? Would you share their contact info with me?

If you are a health care worker, how can you challenge the ways that your professional colleges and employing institutions mandate collusion with police and deny agency to people who are struggling with suicidal impulses?

LESSON SIX:
WE CAN (AND WE MUST)
BUILD A BETTER WORLD

Octavia Butler and adrienne maree brown have brought this lesson to me; we build the world we live in every day, with each of our choices, in each of our relationships. We have not only the ability but the responsibility to reshape it in closer accordance with our values. Can you find ways, micro and macro, to weave these lessons into your practices?

Ask yourself if your choices are in alignment with breaking silences, complexifying dualistic thinking, honouring the wisdom of the body, being in touch with your own consent and the consent of others, and disrupting carceral thinking and carceral systems. What would our communities look like, what would our emergency intervention systems look like, if instead of working so hard to incapacitate suicidal people, we worked toward creating communities that didn't foster so much harm, so that fewer people were in such deep suffering that they imagined dying as their best option? Will you build this world with me?

Ritualizing Queer Care

Blyth Barnow

On the day she died I was sick in bed. A few weeks earlier my illness had been at its worst. I couldn't even keep down small sips of water and had lost almost eighteen pounds in a week. I thought I was dying. I'd managed to fight my way into an appointment at the clinic and demanded an urgent referral to the gastroenterologist, only to find out that "urgent" just meant I could get an appointment in six months instead of eight. So, I went back to bed.

My body was no longer processing food properly. I'd eat a little something, drink a little something, and my body would cramp with severe pain. The doctors told me there was nothing wrong, so it must be stress. Plus, I was fat, so they insinuated it wouldn't hurt to lose some of the weight that was falling off me.

For reasons I will never know, I was feeling a little better that week, which is how I came to spend some of her final days with her. We'd been friends for years, mostly on the community level, both being queer femmes from places outside the Bay Area bubble. We'd been in a burlesque group together and invited each other to our parties. We weren't besties. But we were close enough that I was included in a Facebook message asking people to check in on her because she wasn't doing well.

A few days later she came to my house and we talked for over five hours about grief, relationships, and illness. She tried telling me how bad it had gotten. She'd already been to the hospital by then. She'd wanted to die, and she'd had a plan, so her partner drove her to the hospital so she could check herself in.

The hospital staff left her sitting on a gurney in the hallway for hours. Everybody was just walking right past her, nobody noticing the pain she was in. It made it worse. She told them she was fine and was gonna leave, but they wouldn't let her. So, she slipped out a side door when they weren't looking. They were never looking.

A week later I was with her in a different hospital, one a few counties over, and she'd clearly done her research. The staff seemed kind and there was hope she would actually get the care she needed this time. I'd taken an Imodium and driven over the bridge to get to her. I was terrified they wouldn't let me in, so I stole a stole. You know, one of those things that look like table runners that clergy drape over their shoulders. I snuck into the supply room for the chapel at the seminary I attended and picked out a bright floral stole. It was kind of gaudy, which I knew she would like. I was gonna lie and say I was her chaplain and demand they let me in.

I didn't need it. They let me in. But I was ready anyway. And the stole was beautiful. Just in case. And when people ask me what femme is, I tell them it is something like that. It is stealing what you need from the locked closets of the world and fighting fiercely with all you have for all you love. And yes, we make the fight beautiful because we know that beauty is both an offering and a tool.

A few days later they released her against her objections. She told them she wasn't ready; they told her they'd sign her up for an outpatient program. She died two days later, after she'd gone to do her intake for the outpatient program, and they told her the program was full.

I had plans to see her that afternoon. I was going to drive to her apartment and meet her mother for the first time. But once again my body was uncontained and I couldn't leave my house, so I called her and left a voice mail asking to change our plans. I invited her and her mother to come over to my place and watch *Steel Magnolias* or some other Dolly Parton movie with me. I never heard back. And it hurts me to think that the last thing she may have heard was me saying I was too sick to come to her. Which is to say that our health, or lack thereof, can be a haunting.

I was still in bed when the phone rang about an hour after we were scheduled to get together. Her partner had found her and asked a friend to call and give me the news. I remember the terror and the power of the wail that escaped me and pulled me from bed. I drove over to her partner's house and prayed that they were wrong and that every ambulance I saw held her still living body. But they were right, and she was gone.

I stood with her partner and a friend in the courtyard of their house, surrounded by fragrant flowers and numb with disbelief. I kept staring at her partner's trembling hands. It was the same tremor I would come to recognize in others as the news of her death spread. It was the pulse of coming undone. Behind us the police and coroner moved discreetly behind closed doors. There was nothing for us to do. The finality in the air felt stifling.

I looked over at the angel's trumpet flowers blooming on a nearby shrub. They were pale yellow and beautiful, their blossoms delicate yet assertive. Their scent changed the air around them. I asked her partner and the friend who was comforting them if they wanted a blessing. When they both said yes, I plucked a flower and let the nectar drip onto their wrists, reminding them that they were being held by the vastness and beauty of the universe and they were not alone.

I have learned that when there is nothing left to offer, there is ritual. Some way to hold the moment and honour what is happening. A container we can temporarily surrender our meaning making to.

Something that can take horror and move it beyond us, into a realm more vast and capable of holding it. A mechanism to offer us just a little extra space.

Ritual doesn't have to be elaborate. It just has to be on purpose. There is something sacred in the simple, in using what's elemental and just lying around. It is a reminder that every aspect of our lives is and can be holy. That *we* are holy in the profanity, the ordinariness, of our lives.

The doors behind us opened and several officers wheeled her out on a gurney. Before the coroner took her, I offered her a blessing, too. It was emotional and rambling and imperfect. But it was on purpose. We each picked an angel's trumpet flower, stood beside her, and laid it on her chest. The yellow-white of the flowers against the periwinkle blue of the blanket they'd wrapped her in. A blessing. An adornment. A devastation.

I ended up meeting her mother that night after all, under circumstances far more heartbreaking than I'd imagined. I sat with her in my friend's apartment and made her tea while we waited to hear more from the coroner's office. I turned down every nervous offer she extended to make me food, knowing I couldn't keep it down, and we sat together in untreated grief.

The next few days my body managed to mostly cooperate as I helped to plan her funeral and tended to the personal and collective grief that had broken over everyone I knew. Which is to say that the queer body is capable of superhuman feats when failed by the inhumanity of a medical system that harms us and the people we love.

After the funeral I needed some way to formalize my grief. I decided to enter a forty-day period of mourning. I wanted to honour the devastating nature of her loss while at least trying to care for my own life. During that time, I wore only black, made an altar for her in my bedroom, read poems and prayers in the morning, made doctors' appointments, left a candle lit, and turned down all social invitations. I wasn't following any tradition. I made it up. You are allowed to do that. I followed any small thread that offered comfort or relief and wove those threads together into a daily practice sturdy enough to hold me in my grieving and my illness.

Ritual is simply an offering of respect for the reality of your life. It offers witness when you can't bear to be seen by others. It holds you when you are inconsolable. It connects you to the whole when you feel utterly alone. Ritual has room for complexity and does not require you to tell one story at a time. It offers you care on your terms.

During this time, I continued battling with doctors, trying to get the appointments I needed, trying to get answers. I rarely got to see the same doctor twice. Each appointment I had to describe my symptoms again. I kept having to correct the doctor when they assumed I had diabetes because I was fat. I was continually forced to walk a line between demanding what I needed and being dismissed as hysterical, and I left every appointment without the answers or care I needed. No diagnosis, no follow-up tests, no medication to ease my symptoms, no concern. I'd watched lack of care end my friend's life and couldn't help but worry it would kill me, too.

I wasn't done grieving when that forty-day period of mourning was over. But I was ready for something new, so I decided to enter a forty-day period of living. A time when I did my best to honour the things that made me feel alive, a time to honour the things I loved and make caring for my body my first priority. I made an altar for myself. On it, I put the over-the-counter medications I'd found helpful, a bowl of water to bless myself each morning, my favourite black liquid eyeliner, the only plant I've ever kept alive, a love note from myself, and a collection of tinctures gifted to me by femmes.

My altar was the first and last thing I looked at each day. A reminder that I wanted and deserved to live and live well. A reminder that I am both breakable and resilient. A reminder that my resilience relies on continuous daily care for myself. An affirmation that my real care network is not the medical system but the sick and disabled queers who build community, share skills, and offer what worked for them in similar circumstances.

Queer people rely on ritualizing our worth, even if we don't always name it in this way. We pattern our lives to honour our joy, our humanity, and our capacity to survive. It is how we know we are not alone. It is a reminder that there is something more than the suffering the world has promised us. It is how we grieve our dead and fight for the living. Ritual is our promise that it won't always be this way. Ritual is our reminder that we deserve better now. You can hear it in how we greet each other, see it in how we dress, feel it when we gather. Every day we turn the ordinary into the sacred.

Ritualizing the care I offer myself and others is a way to reclaim power and worth when the "health care" system tries to strip both away. It is an act of love, defiance, and visioning. It is a declaration of dignity and value. It is an assertion that we will not allow this system to kill us without a fight. It is the contrast of a brightly coloured stole against the stark blankness of hospital walls, the soft touch of a flower on your wrist when you are coming undone, the daily witness of homemade altars to living and dying. Ritual care, queer care, is an unbreakable devotion.

Surviving
Together

Zena Sharman

A MASON JAR AND A DREAM

My kid was conceived with the help of a small Mason jar and an infant syringe with the needle removed, mundane implements converted into do-it-yourself (DIY) queer reproductive technologies. Our sperm donor, who lived out of town, would align the timing of his monthly visits to my partner Scout's ovulation cycle. On insemination nights, one of my jobs was to deliver the Mason jar, now holding our donor's semen, to Scout's bedroom and use the syringe to insert it into my partner's body. The first time I helped with an insemination I gushed thanks and praise to our donor as he passed me the jar. He's a quietly kind and generous person and I think my effusiveness might've made him feel shy. Plus, we didn't know each other all that well and it's kind of weird to hand a near-stranger a jar of your jizz, so I kept it low-key after that.

It took a couple of years of on-and-off trying for my partner to get pregnant. Scout was working out of town as the director of a children's summer camp when they peed on a pregnancy test stick and got the positive symbol signifying the "yes" they'd spent so long hoping for. They messaged me with the news soon after. I remember reading their text while standing alone in my kitchen and pausing to gauge my reaction. How *did* I feel now that this was finally happening? I was relieved to notice my dominant emotions were happiness and excitement. Dreaming about having a baby is one thing; actually gestating a brand new human being is another. We'd spent so long existing in hope and hypotheticals I didn't know how I'd feel when it actually happened.

As you read my story, I wonder if you're casting me as the reluctant dad-to-be, the nongestational parent nervous at the prospect of having their first kid. Or maybe you're viewing my partner and me through a halo of homonormativity, a romantic and familiar narrative about two people in love trying to complete their nuclear family by conceiving a much-wanted baby (with a little help from a friend). These stories circulate in our culture; structure our laws, policies, and institutions; and shape our sense of possibilities for what family and parenting can look like.

The story of how I became a parent follows a different narrative. It demands a wider view, a queered way of conceptualizing family, reproduction, and parenting. That's because our kid has four parents, not two, within a family structure rooted in friendship, chosen family, and a purposeful distribution of responsibility and caring labour.

FAMILY AS A TECHNOLOGY OF SURVIVAL

"Family" means many things to queer and trans people. When considered in relation to our families of origin and the families we create, family can be a site of both liberation and oppression. It may be the source of our gravest wounds and where we've done our deepest healing. The family functions as "both a regulatory institution and a site of resistance," dynamics that operate at the level of the nation-state and within communities, as well as within the intimate constellations of people and relationships our families are composed of.[202]

This felt like the hardest chapter to write in *The Care We Dream Of*. Every time I thought I'd figured out what I was trying to say about what family means in relation to queer and trans health, I peeled back another layer of complex, varied, and sometimes conflicting associations, experiences, and histories. People dedicate entire careers to trying to make sense of the family or seeking to reshape or unmake it as an institution. Many of us spend years (and countless hours in therapy) attempting to understand how we were shaped by our experiences of family. What family means to each of us and the extent to which we're free to form families of our own design is entangled with oppression and privilege, dynamics I explore in more detail later in this chapter.

Here, I'm primarily interested in the families queer and trans people intentionally form as adults, families that may or may not include children. Normative concepts like the nuclear family or "next of kin" aren't expansive enough to contain the myriad ways queer and trans people relate to each other and create family. LGBTQ+ people have a long tradition of creating family and caring for each other in the face of harm or rejection by our families of origin, government inaction, or outright aggression, and laws and policies that don't recognize our relationships to each other.

While I may take issue with how discourses of resilience are used in relation to LGBTQ+ health, I hold fast to the truth that resilience is a collective property. As in other communities experiencing systemic oppression, we're practised at fostering relationships grounded in a commitment to our mutual survival. Like all such communities, how we create family, understand and practise kinship, and care for each other are far more expansive than what the state is capable of imagining.

When I think about what family means to me, I think of the creativity, spaciousness, and sheer variety in how the queer and trans community teaches me to imagine and create family. My family is not only who I am connected to through DNA or relationships legible to the state and its laws; it includes my kid and coparents as well as a constellation of other LGBTQ+ people with whom I have intimate and long-standing friendships. In my family, we are in a continual process of choosing each other as we weave and re-weave a sturdy web of care and interdependence together. We are each other's relatives because we make relating a verb; there is a tenderness in these relationships because we tend one another.

It's not always easy or possible to sustain these relationships—it takes work and a commitment to repairing the gaps or tears that form in our shared web. I've experienced the distinctive grief of a friend breakup with someone in my chosen family, an unfixable fissure that still hurts my heart years later. I'm not trying to romanticize these relationships. They're complex, they take effort, and they don't always work out. They're also vital to our health and survival and a source of pleasure, care, and mutual support.

The expansiveness of my queer chosen family contrasts starkly with what I experienced growing up. As a kid, I learned that family was just my mother and me, our connections to the rest of our relatives frayed or fractured by trauma. It was us against the world, though as the child of a disabled single mother on welfare I was conscious of how our ability to survive was subject to the whims of the state and authority figures designated to act on its behalf. I learned the performance of respectability early because I knew it helped keep my family safe from state intervention; as the white child of a white parent, I didn't yet understand how we also were shielded and protected by our whiteness.

I didn't realize it at the time but coming out as queer in my early twenties was the beginning of a massive shift in how I understood and created family, a shift that continues unfolding almost twenty years later. Now that I'm coparenting a toddler in a queer family structure of our own making, my experience of family is stretching and shape-shifting even more. Queerness has given me the ability to create, re-create, and sustain family as an act of love, vibrant creativity, and a commitment to our mutual survival. This experience has offered me healing and changed me on a somatic level as I continue to learn what it feels like to trust in interdependence.

In her book *How We Show Up: Reclaiming Family, Friendship, and Community*, writer and activist Mia Birdsong says, "The places that I've found the strongest, most expansive, boundary-bending, inclusive examples of family and community are among the people who experience the most adversity and oppression."[203] Her book highlights the experiences and practices of Black people, queer people, poor people, and unhoused people in reclaiming and reshaping family. Birdsong celebrates the "breadth and fluidity" of Black families and honours the ways many Black children are raised in constellations of parents, grandparents, aunties, sister-friends, and play cousins.[204] She shares the stories of Mamahouses, collective homes by and for single parents and their children, and Homefullness, a cohousing and social change project for houseless and formerly houseless families and individuals. Throughout her book, she honours the myriad ways queer and trans people form families outside dominant norms. Birdsong affirms the immense power of communities creating family as a form of resistance against all the forces that seek to control or prevent their very existence.

As a queer parent and LGBTQ+ health advocate, I notice myself feeling increasingly compelled by questions of family, kinship, and reproduction and also more acutely aware of how the state attempts to regulate our relationships. While I don't equate family with having or raising children, my experience as a queer parent has pushed me to think more deeply about how to practise interdependence in ways that are deeply inclusive of children and their caregivers. In *Don't Leave Your Friends Behind*, Victoria Law and China Martens observe that when social justice movements and communities fail to support the inclusion of children, they perpetuate and reinforce the belief "that families need to turn back to the dominant system—with all its privilege, lack of privilege, patriarchy, exploitation, inequality, and injustice—to take care of their needs."[205] Countering this dynamic is one of many reasons I want LGBTQ+ communities to be more inclusive of children and their caregivers while also interrogating and disrupting the dominant norm of the nuclear family. Both are part of a larger project of imagining alternative modes of caring for one another.

For many of us, creating our own families can be a technology of survival. As I reckon with the apocalyptic future that often seems to be on the horizon, I wonder what kinds of families and communities we need to create and sustain to help enable our collective survival, flourishing, and liberation. I want to understand and practise ways of relating that create conditions for interdependence and mutual aid within and across generations of queer and trans people.

Independence is a myth that divides us and weakens our collective power, as is the idea we will achieve liberation by politely negotiating with the state or playing by its rules. If we're going to survive, we need to do it together. How can we build on the expertise we already hold through being part of vibrant lineages of queer and trans family-making as a survival technology? What repressive, limiting notions of family, kinship, or reproduction might we need to transform or divest from? As we work toward transformation, how might we strategically navigate the ways the state and the health system attempt to dictate and control who our family can be?

"DON'T TELL ME WHO MY FAMILY IS!"

I once exclaimed, "Don't tell me who my family is!" to a member of the human resources team at an organization where I worked. Years of frustration with how bureaucracies fail to recognize my relationships and webs of care propelled these words out of my mouth. I had to take vacation time when my kid was born because our workplace policies didn't count me as a parent. Since I didn't give birth and am coparenting with three other people, I wasn't eligible for the parental leaves my co-workers (straight or otherwise) in more typical families had access to. Similarly, my partner and I aren't married, and we don't share a home address because we spend half of each week living apart, so our relationship is excluded from workplace policies that would otherwise give them access to additional health benefits through me.

These are small examples of how legal and policy-bound definitions of family perpetuate exclusion and create barriers to resources and supports, underpinned by dynamics of normativity, control, and repression. That repressive quality is evident in the restrictive definitions of family inherent in medicine, the health system, and laws and policies governing access to supports, services, and rights. If you've ever tried to care for or advocate on behalf of a loved one you aren't biologically or legally related to, like a friend or chosen family member, you likely will have encountered multiple barriers in the health system. We often face these barriers during times of crisis, like when someone is seriously ill, injured, or receiving emergency psychiatric treatment, or having a major medical procedure. We also encounter them around birth and death, especially if our loved one is giving birth or dying in an institutional setting like a hospital.

Among LGBTQ+ people, caring for one another is an important way we contribute to our relationships with friends and chosen families as well as a source of "political and social solidarity."[206] However, the caregiving relationships that help queer and trans people stay alive and thriving often go unrecognized or challenged by the state, whose laws and policies are built around limiting assumptions about people's relationship and family structures. The assumption is that everybody has a romantic partner (only one, because monogamy is the default) who they are married to or in a marriage-like relationship with. Marital relationships enshrine a spouse's power to make health care and financial decisions for their partner, have custody of children, and access inheritances, pensions, and other benefits. In many contexts, people's ability to access health care or citizenship is also tied to marriage.

Philosopher Elizabeth Brake describes this phenomenon as "amatonormativity"—that is, the "widespread assumption that everyone is better off in an exclusive, romantic, long-term coupled relationship, and that everyone is seeking such a relationship."[207] Brake points to how this assumption devalues friendships and other caring relationships and has a structuring effect on laws and society. Asexual writer Angela Chen critiques the ways amatonormativity is "woven into our legal rights, creating forms of discrimination that become more and more apparent as people age."[208] In the United States, for example, Chen notes that there are over 1,100 federal laws benefiting couples. Implicit in this is the idea that "the mere presence of romantic feelings" elevates romantic relationships above all others and thus "deserves special protections."[209]

Amatonormativity invisibilizes and excludes people who can't easily locate ourselves in this narrow conceptualization of relationships and families. For example, it leaves out people in polyamorous or nonmonogamous relationships or asexual and aromantic people who build intimate relationships outside of dominant sexual or romantic norms. It also props up state-sanctioned marriage and access to rights and benefits grounded in narrow definitions of family instead of opening up more expansive possibilities for how people might access the resources and supports they need to survive and move freely. While laws in some jurisdictions have changed (for example, to recognize that a child can have more than two parents), normative definitions of family predominate in many of our laws and policies.

This limiting conceptualization of family assumes people have relatives they are legally or biologically related to, whether spouses, siblings, parents, adult children, or others who they can rely on for caregiving and trust to make decisions about their care. The system is designed to prioritize legally recognized family members when assigning these responsibilities. For many queer and trans people whose relationships don't conform to amatonormative stereotypes, this is a form of erasure. For those whose relationships with their families of origin are fractured by trauma, prejudice, or hatred, it can be a form of violence.

If you aren't deemed competent to make your own decisions, you could end up with a person or the state itself designated as your guardian or conservator. When this happens, another person or a government official representing the state is given control over your medical, legal, and financial affairs. This endows them with the power to make decisions about things like where you live and what your daily life is like. Disability advocates have long been critical of these kinds of arrangements. Disabled writer s.e. smith calls them "dehumanizing" and describes how people subject to them are at higher risk of abuse by those responsible for their care.[210] This makes me think of A.H., a disabled woman in British Columbia who in 2019 successfully sued the government health care agency acting as her guardian for detaining her against her will for nearly a year in psychiatric facilities. There, she was physically restrained, cut off from contact with visitors, and denied the ability to go outside for fresh air.[211]

My own family structure is such that I might be in a more vulnerable position if a health care provider or the state had to appoint a decision-maker for me. I'm not married, I'm not especially close with my few living relatives, and my queer chosen family doesn't legally hold the same status as them despite the intimacy of our relationships. Since I don't trust the state to take care of me or respect my wishes, I got the paperwork necessary to legally designate my partner and a close friend as my health care and financial decision-makers. We've had explicit conversations about my health care and end-of-life wishes and what I want to happen to me and my stuff after I die.

This was a defensive, tactical move, one I encourage others in my circles to make. If you're curious about how to do this, start by researching what's legally required where you live (it varies by province or state) and if there are any supports available locally. During the COVID-19 pandemic, for example, the California-based Disability Justice Culture Club held free legal clinics to help disabled people get their health care decision-making paperwork in order. This was part of a wider organizing strategy to resist the harms of ableist medical triage protocols that devalued disabled—and Indigenous, Black, Brown, fat, and older—people's lives.

The way the family functions as a regulatory institution shows up in how family is defined by the state and in our health care system. Implicit in this definition are a whole set of beliefs that value some bodies, lives, and relationships over others. It's important to understand what this means in the context of our everyday lives and communities, as well as how it's shaped the histories that got us to where we are today.

UNDERSTANDING THE PRESENT BY LOOKING TO THE PAST

The first gay fathers group in the United States has its roots in the 1975 San Francisco pride parade. Several months earlier, Jack Latham published an article titled "A Faggot Father Speaks Out" in a gay liberation newsletter, *Gay Sunshine*, where he invited gay fathers in the San Francisco Bay Area to march with him in the upcoming pride parade. As the fathers walked in the parade, others ran out of the crowd to join them, announcing, "You're a gay father, I'm a gay father too!"[212] It was an important moment of community formation at a time when many gay fathers struggled to rectify their identities as gay men and fathers.

Some gay fathers of this era grounded their identities in an explicitly feminist, anticapitalist, gay liberationist politic that sought to challenge the nuclear family. Others sought to project a clean-cut, respectable image of fatherhood in contrast to what one prominent gay father, Bill Jones, described as the "sleaziness" of the pride parade. By the early 1980s, the latter perspective predominated in the increasingly white and wealthy gay fathers movement, which marshalled the language of "family values" in response to the conservative antigay politics of the Reagan era. In his book *Radical Relations*, which chronicles the history of lesbian and gay parenting in the United States between the mid-1940s and early 2000s, historian Daniel Rivers notes, "Later political campaigns for gay and lesbian parental rights and same-sex marriage would inherit this politics of gay familial and domestic respectability."[213]

I offer this history because it feels like a microcosmic example of the power of coming together around shared identities *and* the harms of the wealthier, white LGBTQ+ community's persistent turn toward respectability politics. As I've explored elsewhere in this book, such tactics leave too many of our people behind. When conceiving of the family as simultaneously a regulatory institution and a site of resistance, as Rivers does, I find it helpful to trace some of the historical trends shaping where we are today.

A core argument in Rivers' book is the idea that "one of the foundational notions in American culture is that of the family as by definition heterosexual, along with the inverse idea that queerness is by definition childless."[214] He describes how, in the post–World War II, pre-Stonewall years, many lesbian and gay parents stayed underground out of fear of losing access to their children and being criminalized or incarcerated in a psychiatric facility as punishment for their "deviant" desires.

Beginning in the late 1960s, as more people started publicly coming out, lesbian and gay parents began fighting legal battles for child custody or visitation as their heterosexual ex-spouses or other family members sought to limit or cut off access to their children. These legal fights were buttressed by the idea that queer people were unfit to parent because of the threats our queerness posed to children. In some cases, antisodomy laws were used to criminalize parents, prevent them from seeing their children, limit their ability to participate in LGBTQ+ community activism, or have romantic and sexual relationships with other queer adults.

Researcher and long-time LGBTQ+ parenting activist Rachel Epstein described the climate in Canada during this era as "disheartening, with courts distinguishing between 'good' and 'bad' lesbian mothers (and gay fathers); the good ones being those who were not visible, militant, or sexual."[215] In response, lesbian mothers and gay fathers in the United States and Canada created their own activist groups and organizations, providing legal, emotional, and financial support for child custody cases and offering a much-needed sense of community for people navigating their dual identities as queer people and parents.

Some of these groups made important contributions to subsequent legal advocacy focused on LGBTQ+ domestic and parenting rights. This influenced struggles for domestic partnership recognition and same-sex marriage, as did the experiences of people who were denied access to their sick and dying loved ones or shut out of medical and legal decision-making for chosen family members during the AIDS crisis. Gay liberation–era feminist experiments in alternative family structures and collective child care eventually gave way to more normative family structures, the strategic marshalling of respectability politics by some activists, and growing mainstream representations of LGBTQ+ families.

Lesbian mothers with ties to the women's health movement helped spark the "gayby" boom of the 1980s and 1990s by increasing access to insemination at home and through fertility clinics. For example, three feminist collectives published separate guides to self-insemination in 1979—*Lesbian Health Matters!*, *Woman Controlled Conception*, and *Artificial Insemination: An Alternative Conception for the Lesbian and Gay Community*—with the intention of "helping lesbians and single heterosexual women gain control over their own reproductive decisions" at a time when many fertility clinics deliberately excluded them.[216] For example, Epstein describes how some fertility clinics required lesbians to undergo psychiatric assessments before deciding whether to serve them.[217] My own experiences with DIY home insemination almost forty years later are tied to this lineage of health knowledge reclamation, community skill-sharing, and deliberate circumvention of the health system.

Learning more about this history gave me new insights into my own contemporary experiences of queer parenting and helped me better understand some of the roots of the focus on marriage and family rights that still predominates in many LGBTQ+ advocacy organizations. Many activists and writers have critiqued this focus for how it centres the needs of more privileged members of the LGBTQ+ community and makes harmful concessions to the state. As writer and activist Yasmin Nair writes in the collection *Against Equality: Queer Revolution, Not Mere Inclusion*, the reliance on the marital family structure exemplified by the push for marriage equality allows "the state to mandate that only some relationships and some forms of social networks count."[218]

Nair continues, "A queer radical critique of gay marriage exposes how capitalism structures our notion of 'family' and the privatization of the social relationships we depend on to survive."[219] Unlike a fight for universal health care or the abolition of borders, which would confer life-enabling benefits to many queer and trans people regardless of their relationship status, the fight for marriage equality centred a narrower and more privileged—a.k.a. white, wealthy, and cis—segment of the LGBTQ+ community.

In this context, dominant representations of LGBTQ+ families have "tended to conflate the notion of queer family with normative, two-adult households."[220] Writer Michael Waters connects this to a tendency to represent LGBTQ+ people raising children in a way that's "almost indistinguishable from the straight nuclear family early [gay] liberationists sought to escape."[221] There are many historical and contemporary factors, both political and pragmatic, that drive some LGBTQ+ people into more normative family structures. Those who can conform may derive benefits from doing so, but those benefits often come at the cost of harm to others in our communities.

As we seek to imagine the kinds of family and kinship formations that will help our community survive together, we need to confront the truth that the narrow definition of family that structures our laws, policies, and health system is entangled with racism, eugenics, and social control. Black queer political scientist Cathy Cohen pointed to this fact almost twenty-five years ago when she wrote, "Many of the roots of heteronormativity are in white supremacist ideologies which sought (and continue) to use the state and its regulation of sexuality … to designate which individuals were truly 'fit' for full rights and privileges of citizenship."[222] Cohen illustrates this through examples of how the state limited Black people's ability to marry and how single mothers, teenage mothers, and poor women of colour dependent on state assistance have been stigmatized and demonized.

Cohen called on the queer community to "recognize the links between the ideological, social, political, and economic marginalization of punks, bulldaggers, and welfare queens" as the basis for engaging in progressive, transformative coalition work aimed at shifting power.[223] Her call to action is as relevant today as it was twenty-five years ago. However, the assimilationist tendencies of more privileged members of LGBTQ+ communities and the organizations that advocate on their behalf, along with the entrenchment of survival-of-the-fittest neoliberal inequality, may make answering it even more challenging.

REPRODUCTIVE JUSTICE AND REPRODUCTIVE OPPRESSION

Learning about reproductive justice and reproductive oppression helped me understand more fully how racism and white supremacy, colonialism, ableism, capitalism, and misogyny have sought to regulate and control reproduction and family-making in North America for centuries. As a white cis woman, I'm buffered in many ways from this violence. The reproductive justice movement taught me to ask questions like which people, families, and forms of reproduction are deemed worthy and valuable by the state, and why? Which people, families, and forms of reproduction are deemed wanting, deviant, and in need of control or eradication? Whose bodies, reproductive capacity, communities, and webs of relationships suffer the greatest harm and violence as result? Learning more about the answers to these questions helped me understand that historical and contemporary perspectives on queer family-making and parenting are incomplete if we fail to contextualize them in relation to reproductive justice.

The term "reproductive justice" was invented in 1994 by a group of Black women who were organizing together under the name Women of African Descent for Reproductive Justice against a US government health care reform bill that disadvantaged poor people and women of colour. One of those organizers was Loretta J. Ross, a Black feminist and founding leader of the reproductive justice movement. Ross and her collaborator Rickie Solinger explain that reproductive justice "goes beyond the pro-choice/pro-life debate and has three primary principles: (1) the right *not* to have a child; (2) the right to *have* a child; and (3) the right to *parent* children in safe and healthy environments. In addition, reproductive justice demands sexual autonomy and gender freedom for every human being."[224] As a framework and as a movement, reproductive justice is intersectional and grounded in commitment to human rights. It is rooted in the expertise and experiences of racialized communities whose ability to create and sustain family has been violently suppressed or controlled.

Ross offers a definition of reproductive oppression drawn from the work of Asian Communities for Reproductive Justice (now Forward Together): "Reproductive oppression is the exploitation of our bodies, sexuality, labour, and fertility in order to achieve social and economic control of our communities and in violation of our human rights."[225] As Ross notes, "Through reproductive oppression, you can control entire communities."[226]

Heterosexual, state-sanctioned, monogamous marriage has been used as a tool of settler colonialism, racism, and white supremacy, violently disrupting kinship networks and culture, imposing a binary understanding of gender and sexuality, and dictating access to land, property, citizenship, and health care.[227] As queer scholar Scott Lauria Morgensen observes, "Modern sexuality arose in the United States as a method to produce settler colonialism, and settler subjects, by facilitating ongoing conquest and naturalizing its effects."[228]

Across Turtle Island, Indigenous people's lands and lives were stolen by white settlers, their communities uprooted, and their children taken from them through the genocidal project of residential and boarding schools. Enslaved Black people and their children were treated as property, forced to have children, and then separated from them by white slave owners. Asian and other immigrant communities were prevented from being able to create families for years through racist immigration laws like the Chinese Exclusion Act and laws encouraging people from the global South to move north for child care work, while separating them from their own children and families.

The contemporary child welfare system perpetuates this violence through the disproportionate apprehension of Indigenous, Black, and children of colour and the criminalization of pregnant and parenting people. These same communities are disproportionately affected by mass incarceration and the prison industrial complex, which deliberately weakens or severs family ties, denies incarcerated people access to health care (including reproductive health care), and prevents formerly incarcerated people from accessing housing, employment, and services.[229]

Entire communities are marked as deviant or undesirable and treated as a problem to be eliminated or controlled. Thousands of disabled and Mad people; Black, Indigenous, Latinx, and Asian people; poor people; incarcerated people; and migrants in the United States and Canada have been forcibly sterilized because of eugenicist laws, policies, and medical practices. Disabled people today "are frequently forced to defend their parenting rights and some are barred from having children at all through involuntary and coerced contraception and sterilization."[230] Many LGBTQ+ people face enormous barriers to accessing reproductive and sexual health care, fertility care, and abortion care, limiting their ability to choose if, when, and how they want to become parents.[231]

In a tool kit on queering reproductive justice, Zsea Bowmani and Candace Bond-Theriault remind us, "Those who oppose comprehensive and affordable reproductive health care are often the same forces that want to control what we as lesbian, gay, bisexual, transgender, gender nonconforming, Two-Spirit, intersex, and queer people do with our bodies."[232] This is terrifyingly evident in 2021 as conservative politicians and lawmakers in dozens of US states have introduced antitransgender laws seeking to ban trans youth from accessing gender-affirming health care, some of which seek to criminalize supportive parents and apprehend their trans children.[233] These same politicians and lawmakers also seek to dismantle reproductive health care.

Queer and trans people of colour within the reproductive justice movement have called attention to its heteronormativity and failure to meaningfully integrate a commitment to trans justice, yet they also lift up the power and transformative potential of a movement led by Black, Brown, and women of colour. Trans Afro-Latinx birthworker Lucia Leandro Gimeno emphasized the importance of solidarity in bridging the reproductive justice movement with a trans justice movement that centres the needs of trans women of colour. He wrote, "I don't want any more allies," highlighting the potential for solidarity in developing a shared understanding of the ways trans and cis women of colour's bodies and minds have been targeted by the medical establishment and the police. [234]

As with Cohen's coalitional politic, there is the potential for solidarity as we fight for our rights to comprehensive, affirming, and accessible sexual and reproductive health care, sexual autonomy, gender self-determination, intersex justice and bodily sovereignty, and the ability to create and sustain families in ways that reflect diverse modes of queer and trans forms of kinship.

FROM NEXT OF KIN TO KINFULNESS

African American studies scholar Ruha Benjamin connects reproductive justice to the practice of kinfulness in Black communities: "For the targets of institutionalized kinlessness, reproductive justice requires working deliberately and creatively to engender institutions and environments that foster a *kinful* existence."[235] Writing from a perspective grounded in her experiences of Indigenous kinship, scholar Kim TallBear, a citizen of the Sisseton-Wahpeton Oyate in South Dakota, calls on us to "focus on how to relate more carefully with one another as beings in the world, both within and beyond romantic relations."[236] This network of relations extends to nonhuman and human kin. Elsewhere, TallBear writes that "recognizing possibilities of other kinds of intimacies—not focused on biological reproduction and making population, but caretaking precious kin that come to us in diverse ways—is an important step to unsettling settler sex and family."[237] She connects this critique of normative marriage and family formations to her own practice of, and scholarly work on, critical polyamory.

My own queer four-parent family is rooted in an intentional effort to disrupt a model of parenting rooted in coupledom and romantic love within a nuclear family–like structure. It originated from a deep friendship between my partner Scout and coparent Linden, a queer femme who's long been part of Scout's chosen family. They'd both always wanted children but kept dating people who didn't or weren't ready to have kids, so years ago they committed to coparenting together as friends. By cocreating a family structure based in friendship, they intentionally chose a coparenting dynamic not dependent on an ongoing romantic relationship between them as a couple.

They held fast to this commitment when Linden met her partner Jen a decade ago; their family structure evolved to include her and, when Scout and I became partners several years later, me. This prompted a lot of conversation and self-reflection on how I might fit into their family in ways that felt authentic and sustainable, especially since I'd spent the past decade happily convinced parenting wasn't for me.

We decided on a family structure with lead parents and vice-parents. As the lead parents, Scout and Linden do more of the day-to-day (and night-to-night) caregiving work, carry a bigger share of the mental load of parenting, and have greater decision-making authority over things like our kid's health and development. Jen and I are the vice-parents, a name intended to capture the fact that we have active roles as parents and caregivers but with more flexibility and autonomy than the leads have. The vice-parents do all the everyday parenting stuff—feeding our kid, helping them get dressed, playing with them, putting them to bed—but it's easier for us to tap in and out, and we carry less of the mental load.

Our family structure gives our kid the benefit of four devoted parents, each with our own complementary skills, strengths, and personalities. Plus, the purposeful division of domestic and caring labour means the adults get a lot more help and time off than we would in a two- or one-parent family. I'm grateful for the ways queerness helped us find our way into this family structure, one that allows me to parent in ways that feel accessible, rewarding, and joyful. It's hard work, but it's way easier than it would be if we were doing it as couples or on our own. (It's also why I was able to write this book during a pandemic while coparenting a toddler and holding down a full-time job.)

Becoming part of a four-parent queer family has attuned me in new ways to the challenges inherent in navigating around norms, laws, and policies incapable of conceptualizing families like ours, whether it's in accessing health care, designating our kid's legal parents, writing our wills, or paying our taxes. It's also heightened my awareness of the privileges we hold as white nondisabled middle-class queer people in being able to parent openly in this way without the ongoing threat of state surveillance, intervention, or child apprehension.

As the parent of a young child, I've become more militant about inclusion of children and their caregivers in queer and trans communities. Too few spaces are deeply inclusive of children and the people who care for them, which creates isolation, separation, and the loss of opportunities to forge intergenerational communities. It can push people into dominant systems and family structures we should be working to dismantle. Also, babies, kids, and young people are fucking rad and I have no patience for ageism of any kind.

You don't have to want kids or love kids or even want to spend a lot of time around kids, but you do have a responsibility to cocreate a community that's welcoming to them. If you've ever wondered where your queer and trans friends with kids disappeared to, consider asking them how you might show up for each other in ways that create more possibilities for mutual care and support. Another good place to start is by reading books like Victoria Law and China Martens's *Don't Leave Your Friends Behind* or Mia Birdsong's *How We Show Up*, both cited earlier in this chapter. As explored elsewhere in this book, our responsibility to cocreate accessible, intergenerational communities must also centre the needs and priorities of Black, Indigenous, and people of colour, poor people, disabled people, and queer and trans older adults.

Ten years ago, I married my former partner. It was a decision grounded in the love I felt for them and also in fear: both my own fear of abandonment and fear of what might happen if one of us got sick or hurt and couldn't advocate for the other. Shortly before we got engaged, I watched a documentary at my local queer film festival that told the stories of LGBTQ+ people who'd been barred from making decisions for or even visiting their critically ill, injured, and dying partners. I remember sitting in the dark movie theatre, the smell of popcorn in the air, tears streaming down my face as I imagined myself in their place.

I'm not married anymore (hello, fellow gay divorcees) and I'm still afraid of what might happen if the state tries to block me from caring for the people I love in times of crisis. What's different now is I don't think marriage is the solution to my fears, nor is taking refuge in the nuclear family. In saying this, I'm not trying to be prescriptive: each person reading this has a set of choices and possibilities available to you about your family and relationship structures. The limitations and/or expansiveness of those choices and possibilities are directly tied to the dynamics of privilege and oppression explored throughout this chapter.

What I'm trying to get at is that how we relate to one another and form families are both intensely personal and highly politicized decisions, ones that have implications for queer and trans people's individual and collective well-being. Any solution that privileges the needs of rich white cisgender LGBTQ+ people is inherently incomplete and fundamentally harmful. It's essential we ground this work in reproductive justice, decolonization, disability justice, economic justice, and migrant justice.

My own experiences have made me curious about the possibilities inherent in creating, experimenting with, and advocating for alternatives to normative family structures in ways that are spacious enough to encompass the diverse ways we relate to each other. I wonder what it might look like to commit to collectivity, both in how we coexist in our communities today and in how we dream and build for the future. As I imagine future forms of kinship, I dream of a world where the kinds of families we create are expansive and sturdy enough to hold us all.

Sowing Seeds from My Ancestors, Planting Seeds for My Descendants

Interview with Sean Saifa Wall

Sean Saifa Wall (he/him/his) is a Black queer intersex activist, visual artist, and rising scholar. He is a Marie Skłowdoska-Curie fellow examining the erasure of intersex people from social policy in Ireland and England (intersexnew.co.uk). Saifa is committed to racial equity and a radical vision of bodily autonomy for intersex folks. As a cofounder of the Intersex Justice Project (intersexjusticeproject.org), a grassroots initiative by intersex people of colour, he is determined to end intersex genital surgery in the United States. Our conversation reflects Saifa's deep commitments to intergenerational activism, fostering intersex community, and creating a more just health system.

Zena: What does intersex justice mean to you?

Saifa: Intersex justice is an evolving ideology that looks at how intersex issues interact with different liberatory struggles. When I think about intersex justice, I think about the ways it intersects with Black liberation, trans liberation, and reproductive justice. How does it tap into, speak to, and be informed by these other liberation movements?

For me, the heart and the crux of intersex justice is recognizing the harm that has befallen intersex individuals who are born with atypical bodies and have been harmed by the medical establishment. But it's also about allowing people who are intersex to be in their bodies and to be free, whether or not they've been harmed. People have a right to live with dignity and be free from stigma and shame.

The idea of reparations is another critical component of intersex justice, in the form of apologies from institutions that have caused harm, recognizing the harm that has been done and making very specific amendments to address the harm. When I envision what the implementation of intersex justice would look like, I think about things like psychological support for parents and free medical care for people who have been harmed to have elective surgeries they choose.

Zena: What does intersex justice look like in practice, both at the level of a whole system and at the level of relationships between patients and health care providers or within families?

Saifa: For me, the bare bones of intersex justice are a radical love and an acceptance of intersex people. When that love and acceptance present, people recognize that variations exist and not all bodies are the same, and everyone deserves to be treated with the same level of dignity and respect.

The implementation of intersex justice in a medical setting would be practitioners who listen and who recognize they have a patient who may have been harmed by the medical establishment. It's patient-informed health care where medical providers understand each person has a body of wisdom inside of them and they should listen to that wisdom.

Intersex variations are often presented by medical providers as disorders, problems, or abnormalities. We need to normalize those variations. Parents and families put so much trust in medical providers. What would it be like if doctors were to say, "Your baby has these differences. It's not life-threatening. They will be okay." And then the doctors work with the parents to create a treatment plan that really centres the child and doesn't include surgery on that child, because surgery reinforces the idea that something is wrong, that there's a pathology that needs to be addressed or fixed.

What would it look like if providers and parents had these conversations in a way that didn't come from a place of pathology? There's often this idea that parents of intersex children are vulnerable to being influenced by medical providers to consent to surgery on their child, and I think that's partly true, but I also think bias exists because we're all shaped by the gender binary.

Part of loving and accepting an intersex child in a context of intersex justice is parents willing to confront their internalized biases about gender and gender roles. The gender binary hurts everyone—intersex people, trans people, non-trans people. When I think long-term about what intersex justice could be, I imagine intersex people existing in an ecosystem, an orbit, a stratosphere of connections that really see them, affirm them on their path, and push them along on their journey in a way that is not stigmatizing or pathologizing and that actually respects the whole of the individual.

Zena: I love the idea of the stratosphere. I keep picturing a much more expansive container or web of support and radical love. I see you putting that commitment and that radical love into action very deeply in what you do and how you move through the world.

Saifa: It's definitely a practice, for sure.

Zena: Speaking of your practice, for several years you and your comrades at the Intersex Justice Project (IJP) have been deeply in the work of calling on Chicago's Lurie Children's Hospital to stop performing surgeries on intersex children. What has this campaign taught you about strategies for holding the health system accountable for medical violence against intersex people?

Saifa: The idea for this campaign was like a meeting of the minds. Pidgeon Pagonis, who's an intersex person and social justice activist in Chicago, was harmed at Lurie Children's Hospital. When the hospital was undergoing a renovation, Pidgeon did a photo series in front of it where they made statements like "I was harmed here."

In 2015, I submitted a funding proposal to a foundation proposing protests in three different cities. One would be at Johns Hopkins where John Money practised, one would be at the Medical University of South Carolina, where MC, a Black intersex kid, was mutilated while in foster care, and the third was Chicago because Pidgeon had roots there. I didn't end up getting the funding, but we decided to do a protest anyway.

We were talking about it and I said we need to have a banner that says, "Intersex children are harmed here." And Pidgeon came up with the hashtag #EndIntersexSurgery. IJP released our first statement in 2016. It was a statement for justice by intersex people of colour. We were reclaiming our place in the movement.

Before IJP was a thing, Pidgeon and I both felt that intersex people of colour, the labour of Black people, femmes, disabled people, and other marginalized communities always gets overlooked in social justice movements. And the representation of intersex was so white. We needed to create a place for intersex people of colour to feel safe and assert themselves as leaders within the movement.

The strategy behind Lurie was that, if we could get one hospital to fold, it would set up a domino effect for hospitals. It would set a precedent that intersex people who have been harmed by these institutions will stand up for themselves and defend the rights of other intersex people. We were harmed by this institution and we took it to the streets, just like our ancestors did, like in 1996 when intersex activists protested the American Academy of Pediatrics conference.

We had a strategy where, with time, persistence, and building relationships across movements and with different people who supported us, we would be victorious. Lurie issued an apology and said they will stop doing surgeries. They put a moratorium on these surgeries for six months so they could produce a white paper on it. Six months is long enough for the surgeries to stop but not so long that they can dodge accountability. Now that Boston Children's Hospital has ended clitoroplasties and vaginoplasties, Lurie is reconsidering its position on these surgeries.

In the aftermath of the Lurie campaign, a journalist asked me about its emotional toll on me. It was the first time I was forced to reckon with the huge emotional toll of sharing my story over and over. I know what I'm fighting for and I have a deep conviction around it. We're fighting for justice and for sovereignty over our bodies in a system that says we're not normal and need to be surgically corrected.

This campaign is the seed. I'm planting seeds for future generations of activists. Whatever they want to do with the harvest is up to them—how they choose to redistribute the seeds, save them, throw them away, that's their choice.

Zena: Can you tell me more about how the leadership of intersex people who are Black and people of colour has shaped the Lurie hospital campaign and your experiences of organizing inside of it?

Saifa: The IJP isn't a nonprofit. That means we don't have the kind of deadlines or have to make up numbers the way you have to with other kinds of funding, like "Oh, we served five people." We also had support from community; there are people who have given very generously from their own pockets and allowed us to share our story on different platforms. I wanted IJP to have a very radical politic, and because we weren't confined in the ways we would be in a traditional nonprofit structure, it allowed us to take risks.

I did a lot of the writing for IJP, and in that writing I drew lines between intersex justice and other movements so intersex issues don't continue to exist in a silo. I wanted people to see that the state violence that happens to intersex people can happen to anyone. If we're sterilizing people and allowing hospitals and the state to sanction people's bodies, what else can happen?

Intersex activism has made the conversation on medical accountability real. How do we hold accountable practitioners who have never been held accountable for their actions? How do we do that in a public forum?

For me, as a Black intersex person, I see the ways in which the state has harmed my body but also has harmed my family. Centring Blackness in intersex work was never up for debate for me. It's always been there, so I have always prioritized the leadership of Black people and people of colour.

I think sometimes, especially in these moments in the wake of George Floyd and other state-sponsored, extrajudicial killings of Black people, there's this rush that happens, right? Liberal and progressive people say, "We need a Black person! Find a Black person now!" And for me and IJP, it's not just about finding a Black person; it's about cultivating their leadership over time. That was and still is my vision for IJP.

I am deeply committed to this radical vision of IJP where Black and intersex people of colour have a home. I think IJP represents the promise of what Black and intersex people of colour can contribute to this conversation around freedom, liberation, and taking back what was taken from us.

Zena: Many intersex people have experienced medical violence and violation of their bodily autonomy, sovereignty, and consent when accessing health care. What would it look like to offer intersex folks care and healing in a way that really honours and loves their intersex bodies?

Saifa: I recently had a conversation with an intersex person in Bangladesh who experienced six surgeries when they were younger, some of which were exploratory so medical providers could see the inside of their anatomy. This person identifies as male and people ask them now, "Why don't you have top surgery?" And at this point in their life, their response is, "I don't want any more surgery!"

When we were talking, I asked them about their vision for Bangladeshi intersex folks. They told me they want a safe house for intersex people who don't have family or support. That stayed with me. What does it mean to keep us safe? What does it mean for intersex people to feel safe in their bodies, in their homes, and with medicine? How can we take those steps for intersex people to feel at home?

People talk a lot about the idea of being at home in your body. But when your house gets robbed, it feels like your home has been violated and desecrated by someone you don't know. To feel safe in your home and neighbourhood again, you have to go through a process of connecting with them. But some people can't; some people move. For intersex people, I think the question is how can your body become home? How do you feel safe in your home again?

One of the liberatory models I use is somatic awareness. It's not a perfect process and I don't expect it to work for everyone, but it has helped me come back to my body in some ways. And there are still so many things I'm learning about my body. Black people, people of colour, Indigenous folks, disabled folks, intersex folks—so many of us experience oppression in and on the body. One modality of liberation I've used is to see where oppression lives in my body and get it out, or address it, confront it, or look at it.

I want people to feel at home in their bodies again and to have this deeply felt sense that they are normal and whole, despite what happened to them. I like the idea of collage because you take different elements and make something new. For intersex people who have been violated, what would it look like to take these pieces of yourself that have been desecrated and create something new?

Intersex surgeries exist in rape culture. There's this idea that this thing is done to you and that's it, you're just left with the violation. Intersex justice says no, we get to reclaim what has been done to us and what has been taken away from us. Our narrative isn't decided for us; we get to tell our own narrative and hold our perpetrators accountable.

Zena: In a piece of writing you shared with me, you wrote that intersex justice "affirms bodily integrity and bodily autonomy as the practice of liberation." Will you tell me more about the embodied connections between intersex justice, the practice of liberation, and how justice and liberation feel in your Black intersex trans body?

Saifa: Intersex justice frees us all. It exposes the bias that exists against intersex people and holds doctors accountable for how they treat people. Bias harms different people within medicine. That kind of bias contributed to the disproportionate number of Black people who died during the COVID-19 pandemic; it also shows up in how some medical students and health care providers believe the racist myth that Black people have thicker skin or don't feel pain in the same ways white people do.

I had a colonoscopy yesterday and the nurse, who was white, stabbed me with the needle while she was looking for a vein. She said, "Oh, your skin is so tough." And I was just like, "My skin is not tough." I have very soft skin. She was dismissing how she poked me in two places while she was searching for a vein and it hurt, and she was just not attuned to that.

When I share my story as an intersex activist, it's a way of showing what the state can do to us. And if we don't say something, if we don't stand up, it can happen to any one of us. I think a big parallel is people being disappeared at protests. There have been people who have been snatched up in our streets for years and deported, but because we don't see migrant people as the same as us, we're just like, "Oh, it's those people over there." We don't have a reason to care until it happens to us. If we allow the state to harm the very vulnerable among us, the state will start to harm all of us.

When I think about why I do this work, why I fight, it's so that little children don't have to endure what I did, so that they might be able to grow up and make decisions about their bodies that feel good to them. I recently met a Black child in Georgia who was born with an intersex variation. Intersex justice is my experience of holding this child and thinking, *This is what makes this work important.* I've stayed in this work to have moments like this, when this child is not bullied by a provider who's telling her mother that her child's body is a problem or something wrong.

There are moments when I've felt very defeated and tired, and I want to give up. Then I'll receive a message from someone who says, "What you did changed my life. Keep doing your work because it's saving lives." I do this work to prevent future harm.

Zena: When you were talking to me about the experience of holding that Black child, I had a visceral feeling of what it's like to hold a baby in my arms or have a kid sit in my lap, the beautiful weight of their being. It's not about just one child, and also it is, in the sense that you have helped shape the trajectory of this child by protecting her from harm. That's not a one-time intervention; it's something that echoes across time. Your work really matters, is what I'm saying. And I'm sure it's really fucking exhausting a lot of the time.

Saifa: Yeah, it sometimes just feels like you're beating your head against the wall. I'm convinced there are some pediatric urologists who are psychopaths, because despite the protests of so many intersex activists who have said the same thing for decades, the resistance is so mighty. And the ask is so, so minimal—just to delay genital surgery until a person can decide what to do with their own body.

Zena: It makes me think about the mindset doctors get trained inside of, starting in medical school. Research shows people become less empathetic as they move through their medical training, and burnout contributes to biased decision-making in medicine. The mindset is so deep, and the entire system is embedded inside of capitalism, ableism, and white supremacy in a way that keeps replicating these violent modes of care and a construction of expertise that serves so few people.

I'm not writing off medicine entirely—I know people who have had treatments that have saved their lives or who rely on western medicine for their ongoing well-being—but the mindset and system it's inside of is founded in so many fundamentally violent and oppressive assumptions. How do we upend that? How do we change the system from both inside and outside of it?

Saifa: For real! Yesterday, when I had the colonoscopy, it was an elective treatment. I consented to it, and I was very happy from start to finish. I knew I was in good hands. When I talked with the surgeon, I disclosed to her that I have an intersex variation and she was so gracious. She said, "Well, Mr Wall, that's in your file. I already know that." And I'm like, great! Love it!

When I broke my right wrist back in 2017, I sought out the help of a surgeon who had razor-sharp precision. When I went back to him for a follow-up visit and he took the X-rays, he was marvelling at his own work. That's what I was looking for, that's what I wanted. In those moments, I'm so appreciative of medicine. This is where allopathic medicine really shows up.

The problem is when intersex is classified as a pathology. We're not a pathology, disease, or disorder; we're not these beings that need to be fixed. Our bodies are fine. We don't need surgery to make us look more "typical," whatever the fuck that means. For me, part of being an intersex activist is developing a very razor-sharp focus on where we need to address the source of harm.

A lot of the harm is being perpetrated by pediatric urologists who are bent on this ideology where there are "typical" bodies. The underlying message is, if your body is atypical, you're not deserving of peace. You're not deserving of bodily integrity because your body needs to be fixed in this conservative, stifling, and oppressive way.

Zena: What are your freedom dreams? When you dream into a more just and liberated world, what does it look and feel like? How does it smell? What does it sound like? How does it feel in your spirit? Who's there with you?

Saifa: I recently had a friend who passed. She was my first love. We met in an internet chat room, how the queers used to do back in the day. We would write letters back and forth and I visited her a couple of times. We broke up because we were literally children, but we stayed friends over the years. We had a conversation a few months ago and I thought her colon cancer had gone into remission, but she died from cancer recently. She was thirty-nine, so young.

When I think about her, when I think about people on the other side who have become ancestors, when I get down to the bare bones of it, I really want my people to just live. My sister who passed away from diabetes suffered so much before she died. They amputated a few of her toes. She was blind. I don't want my people to suffer anymore.

Right now, we exist in this realm of social media. There's this psychic violence that happens every day when someone's death is broadcast. I can see how my heart feels heavy. I can see the fear and anxiety in my friends' faces and feel this collective weight in my community. Even if it didn't happen to you, it could happen to you. That's the psychic violence.

When I think about the turn of the twentieth century when you had extrajudicial murders of Black people by lynching, even though the number of people who were lynched was small compared to the number of Black people who existed at that time, the psychic violence was profound. This may not be you, but it can happen to you. This harms hundreds of thousands of people, even when a few thousand are killed.

I want my people to have peace of mind and peace in their hearts. I want them to have joy—unapologetic, radical joy. I want them to laugh with each other, eat with each other, flirt, fuck, just have that zesty juiciness of life without fear. We need to cultivate these spaces of joy, especially in this moment of heightened, violent white supremacy. This will carry our vision of liberation forward.

When I think about my ancestors, I'm not too far removed from slavery. My grandmother's grandparents were enslaved, possibly her parents were enslaved. My mom's father's parents were enslaved. My mom was born during Jim Crow. I am not far removed from this legacy at all. Because of this legacy, the trauma lives in our bodies. We have existed under this cruel and oppressive system for so long.

What does it look like for Black people to feel safe, to be able to connect with the dirt? When I think about home, ancestors, and legacy, there's something about putting my hands in the dirt, feeling this dirt, crumbling, this rich, moist dirt crumbling between my fingers, you know? Because I know one day that that's the place I will return to.

What does it mean to actually feel my hands, feet, and toes digging into the soft earth? I want my people to know what that feels like. There's something so divinely and uniquely human to be able to touch this thing that's all around us. It's part of us and will one day be our resting place.

Zena: Returning to the theme of intergenerationality, what have you learned from your ancestors? What are the gifts that you want to pass down to your descendants? I've heard you talk about legacy before, including in this conversation, and the idea of sowing seeds for your descendants. When you think across those timelines and relationships, what do you dream into? What do you want your legacy to be as you do this work in your lifetime?

Saifa: I think a lot about legacy because it's an absolute truth. You live and you die, period. While we're here on this earth, we have work to do. I believe part of my work is to avenge the suffering of my ancestors and to notice the seeds they planted for me. I need to look at the harvest I get to reap because of the seeds my ancestors planted for me.

Even in moments of brutality, when Black people were not even considered human, my people were still able to cultivate joy. People were able to sit under a tree, make dolls or quilts, laugh together, sing, or go to church. They found home in each other. When emancipation was upon them, they looked for their loved ones. There's something so profound that people, even in the face of white vigilante terrorism, were able to cultivate joy in the sense of community. They were able to find home within each other and on the land.

When I think about my intersex ancestors, when I think about my two uncles who have already passed, I think about how I can be bolder for them in ways they couldn't be bold. There were ways they had to hide, to talk about their intersex bodies in whispers. How can I be bold for them? How can I avenge their suffering so their spirits can rest?

I want their spirits to know I'm reaping this harvest because they laid those seeds for me. They did what they could to survive, but they planted the seed so I can know that they should not have suffered, and my descendants will not suffer. As I talk to the young people who are coming up, to the young people who are healing, I'm just like, I'm here, I have always been here, and I will be here until I am here no more.

I ask them, "What do you need from me? What do I need to say, what do I need to do so that you will be okay? What do I need to do to pass the torch so that you can continue sprinting?" There is no finish line. We're just passing it forward, generation by generation.

As I get older, this conversation about legacy always moves me because I've already had dreams of the other side. I've had dreams about the eternal rest of death. They say one of your ancestors, one of your family members, greets you on the other side. I've seen the other side and there's something about it that's just like, my soul is at rest and I don't feel scared. I don't feel like I'm fighting. I'm walking with my dad and my mom and my grandmother and all these people that have transitioned, you know? And I'm still left here, carrying on the fight for them by telling their stories. And when I die, someone will tell my story.

I want to feel like I leave these seeds everywhere, whether I write it, speak it in interviews or protests or whatever; I leave the seeds so that someone who doesn't know me, who I will never know, some organisms, some aliens, can find the seeds I've planted and say, "This is what I've been looking for."

I know that at some point my journey here is gonna end and I will just go back, you know, I will just go back, go ahead, go wherever my next journey is. I feel like they'll be able to take up the mantle and continue fighting, but also continue loving, continue fucking, continue living their best goddamn life because they fucking deserve it. 'Cause life ain't all about the goddamn struggle. Life is also about living and living well.

THE CARE WE DREAM OF

Hungry for Possibilities

Too Many Beloved Dead, Too Few Elders

Zena Sharman

At my fortieth birthday party I told the friends gathered in my living room that I wanted to get old with them, *really* old. And I do. I want to be a badass old femme radical grandma with tattoos and a garden, and I want my friends and loved ones to get really old alongside me. I dream of living with my queer chosen family in an intergenerational community where we take care of each other, have fun together, and share what we have, where no one feels isolated and everyone has enough. I dream of dying at home as an old woman, surrounded by people I love, in a way that feels sacred to me.

At a broader level, I dream of a world where all LGBTQ+ people are able to live long, full lives in interdependent, intergenerational, accessible communities where everyone has what they need to thrive, and no one is living in poverty or isolation. I dream of queer and trans communities with an abundance of older people and elders in them, and for there to be more relationship-building, knowledge sharing, and mutual aid across and within generations of queer and trans people.

My dreams reflect what I hope aging could look like for me. But when I get really honest with myself, I have to admit they're also about my deepest fears. I dream in an attempt to ward off my nightmares about being old, poor, alone, and stuck inside a heteronormative institution. I fear living in a long-term care facility where my independence is limited by adherence to an institution's strict rules and rigid schedule, and where I don't feel free to express my identity as a queer femme. The COVID-19 pandemic made my nightmares worse as I watched how it exacerbated the already deplorable living and working conditions inside these facilities, leading to hundreds of thousands of deaths among residents and staff in Canada and the United States.[238]

This essay is an attempt to face my nightmares in the spirit of dreaming into something different, not just for me but for every queer and trans person who's lucky enough to get old. Because I want us to think that getting old *is* lucky. I want us to know we *can* get old; that it's a possibility that's actually available to us. I want us to know that we don't have to get old alone and that we can be loved and cared for in intergenerational, interdependent communities during all the stages of our lives. I want us to know that we're free to be our full selves as we age, that getting older doesn't mean going back in the closet or dulling our glorious shine.

To do this will require us to reckon with some of the things that get in the way of our ability to imagine different possibilities about aging: what it means to give and receive care in a context of heteronormativity, cisnormativity, and neoliberalism; how ageism shows up in LGBTQ+ communities; and learning how to practise interdependence. It also means changing our expectations and imagining different possibilities about aging. Despite the eldercare industry's (and some LGBTQ+ advocates') emphasis on creating more inclusive, LGBTQ+-friendly institutions, rainbow nursing homes aren't the answer. I want transformation, both for me and the generation of people I'm aging alongside, and for the generations that come after us.

DREAMING OF QUEER AGING (AND FEARING THE NIGHTMARE OF NEOLIBERALISM)

Aging has been on my mind a lot more often since I turned forty, a milestone that got me thinking about what it means for me to get older as a queer person. How many years do I have left, and is this actually the middle of it all? I realize there are no guarantees when it comes to my life expectancy—anything can happen, and it always does—but there's something about this moment that's got me fervently hoping for more. It's partly because I saw my mom die at sixty-six, an age that feels younger and younger the closer I get to it. But it's also because I'm hungry for more life. There's so much I still want to learn, and so much more I want to do. I'm not done living yet.

I have a personal stake in how our community perceives aging and how we treat older people. I'm getting older right now in a way more apparent to me at mid-life than when I was younger—and I want a future that looks different from what I see around me. When I was in graduate school, I started doing academic research on home care in Canada. I remember reading studies that talked about how older women were particularly vulnerable to ending up living alone in poverty. A lifetime of unpaid caregiving work and gendered wage gaps for paid work, along with a longer average life expectancy, leaves many women poor and isolated in old age. That research scared me; it felt like a window into my possible future. I didn't have a family safety net to catch me; there wouldn't be an inheritance to cushion me if I fell. My mom was already an older single woman living in poverty. I had no reason to believe my future would be different from hers.

I started saving for retirement in my twenties because I was afraid and because I was convinced there would be no one to take care of me when I got old. But it's been more than fifteen years since then and I'm still afraid, more so now after studying a broken eldercare system as a researcher, then watching my mom live inside it for six years before she died. She had a rotating cast of underpaid care workers coming through her home, their jobs structured in such a way where they could only provide the bare minimum of care. As someone without siblings, the alternative was for me to quit my job, uproot my life, and move across the country to care for my mom. I couldn't do that, so care provided by the state was our only option. Her home care workers did the best they could, but their working conditions and the rationing of care meant it was never enough, and my mom was fiercely resistant to the idea of living in an institution. She wanted to stay at home for as long as possible, and she did, right up until the last week of her life.

My mom and I were lucky to live in a country with publicly funded health care, but that care was insufficient because the system is built on the assumption that individuals exist inside of heteronormative nuclear family structures. It's a system that relies on an inexhaustible supply, both real and imagined, of unpaid or underpaid feminized (and often classed and racialized) care work that's supposed to fill the gaps created by neoliberalism.

Many queer and trans people live inside those gaps. Often alienated from our families of origin, queer and trans people create our own family structures and care for each other in a context of relationships that may not be recognized by the state. That kind of recognition matters when it limits our ability to visit, make decisions on behalf of, or access resources for our loved ones. As Liz Bradbury, an older adult and advocate for LGBTQ+ older adults, points out, "the adult children model of care is so ingrained into senior care protocol" that many care professionals can't think beyond it.[239] She calls on professionals to stop assuming that adult children or family will be available to care for LGBTQ+ people as we age.

And while LGBTQ+ people are more likely to provide informal care to our loved ones, not everyone *has* chosen family they can rely on for caregiving. This has implications for older adults' ability to get the care they need. Bradbury notes that mainstream society creates the conditions for isolation among LGBTQ+ older adults, yet caregiving protocols for our community assume everyone has chosen family to rely on for caregiving or that they have the capacity to create those relationships in old age.[240] She calls for the creation of programs that expressly support LGBTQ+ older adults to build families of choice. In an essay on care webs and creating collective access, Leah Lakshmi Piepzna-Samarasinha points out not everyone wants their friends as caregivers, which underscores why we also need more and better options for high-quality, dignified, free and affordable care provided by paid caregivers working under conditions that support them to flourish alongside the people they care for.[241]

Since queer and trans people across the lifespan are more likely to live in poverty, including in old age, we may be more reliant on government for housing, income support, and professional caregiving.[242] As researcher Hannah Kia points out, LGBTQ+ older adults have a greater likelihood of being "disciplined and vilified, not only for their non-normative sexualities and gender identities, but also as a category of 'dependent subjects' within the context of a neoliberal welfare state that often disciplines expressions of reliance in older adults."[243] Relying on government support in a context of neoliberalism is dangerous because a neoliberal state doesn't operate on the basis of an ethic of care but rather an aggressive individualism rooted in capitalism, ableism, cisheteropatriarchy, and white supremacy.

To be poor and dependent on the state means having fewer choices, or none at all. Wealth buys options, which is fundamentally inequitable. As housing advocate Janet Torge put it when describing her vision of publicly funded, community-led "radical resthomes" for older adults, "if you have lots of cash, investments and pension, you CAN create a lifestyle of your choosing ... but people like me will never be able to join them, savings-challenged and pension-less that we are."[244] I want us to change that.

QUEERING TIME AND LIVING INSIDE THE PARADOX OF QUEER AGING

Queerness and transness bend time; we're both younger and older at once. Our lives as LGBTQ+ people are shaped by the specific ways we relate to time and resist normative conceptualizations of the life course. As theorist Jack Halberstam writes, "queer temporality disrupts the normative narratives of time that form the base of nearly every definition of human."[245] We remain youthful through developmental trajectories that may include more than one puberty or adolescence. We progress through our lives in ways that don't necessarily map onto the milestones and stages that constitute typical narratives of adulthood and aging. Nonbinary age activist Ryan Backer likens this sequence of normative achievements—things like going to university or college, getting a job, dating, getting married, buying a home, having kids, retiring, having grandkids—to an escalator that ends in the perception of an "accomplished" life.[246] As LGBTQ+ people, we might move through those stages later or not at all; we chart our own paths as we queer time.

Yet it sometimes seems like queer and trans folks get older sooner than other people. In her essay "Where Did She Go?," Kai Cheng Thom writes about her experiences mentoring other trans femmes. She writes, "I started mentoring people in my early twenties and it wasn't really a choice—there was no one else to do it."[247] Thom's experiences are shaped by the many forms of transmisogynistic and racist violence that cut short trans women's lives, particularly among those who are Black, Indigenous, or people of colour. They also resonate with wider patterns I observe across queer and trans communities:

many of us become mentors earlier in our lives through how we form families and share knowledge essential to our survival. We practise mutual aid as we become each other's role models.

When I think about aging in the queer and trans community I come up against a set of ideas that feel paradoxical to me: Many of us don't believe we'll live long enough to get old, our sense of the future foreshortened by violence and trauma. We don't plan for the future because we don't believe it will come, but what happens to us when it does? Those among us who survive don't know how to get old. Some of us hope to live long lives, but most of us are afraid of getting older. We want to live, and we also fear aging and dying for so many reasons wrapped up in how ageism and ableism devalue, infantilize, and desexualize the body/minds of people who are older, disabled, or both.

We're afraid of losing the social value, desirability, freedom, and independence that are associated with youth, of being isolated or institutionalized. Do a Google image search for "LGBT people" and you'll find photo after photo of young-looking people wrapped in rainbow flags. Gay cruising apps like Grindr have been criticized for ageism, with some users putting age limits or "no old men" in their profiles, and research has shown a link between internalized age-ism and depression in gay men.[248] As Ela Przybylo argues in *Asexual Erotics*, "ageism is a politics of disposability, a will to make disappear those deemed discardable by society."[249] She continues, "Older adults, held as abject, leaky, dying, and thus as toxic to the spirit and energy of the population more broadly, are forbidden from enjoying their bodies or from forming alliances with other bodies." Learning how to live to get old means unpacking this.

QUEERNESS AND THE LIMITS
OF INTERDEPENDENCE

A defining characteristic of the LGBTQ+ community is our ability to foster kinship networks outside the families we're born or adopted into. Queer community taught me new ways to build relationships and create family; it's made me more interdependent and more able to trust in interdependence. Sins Invalid defines interdependence as "The state of being dependent upon each other."[250] Mia Mingus elaborates on this idea in a blog post on interdependency:

> Interdependency is both "you and I" and "we." It is solidarity, in the best sense of the word. It is inscribing community on our skin over and over and over again. It is truly moving together in an oppressive world towards liberation and refusing to let the personal be a scapegoat for the political.[251]

Interdependence in queer and trans communities can take many forms, like people circulating financial resources to support community members during times of crisis or raising funds to help someone access the health care they need. It can look like care collectives, text check-ins with a friend who's feeling suicidal, deliveries of meals to new parents or to a community member recovering from gender-affirming surgery; it can look like a femme clothing swap, a child care co-op, or a medication exchange.

We are interdependent in many ways, our chosen families and communities woven together in webs of support and care. We take care of each other. Except when we don't, and that's when we confront—or fall into—the gaps between our idealized vision of the LGBTQ+ community and the reality that many people don't have the support and care they need. For example, in an article about long-term survivors of the AIDS crisis in San Francisco, journalist Erin Allday tells the storis of several HIV-positive gay men in their sixties and seventies.

They never planned for a future they didn't believe would come and now live in isolation and poverty, feeling abandoned and forgotten by the gay community, their circumstances worsened by gentrification and lack of access to services and supports.[252]

Interdependence isn't just a romantic ideal; it's a practice, and when we practise something, we need to keep doing it over and over again, even when it's difficult. As I get older the limitations of how we currently practise interdependence become more obvious to me, as do how ageism and ableism show up in our communities. I've been out as queer for almost twenty years. During that time, and still, my social circles have often consisted of people similar in age to me, give or take around five to ten years. As my peers and I get older, many of us have become less involved in the events, parties, and bar culture that can seem so central to queer life. We like to go to bed early now, or we're tired, or we can't get child care, or we got sober, or we listen to our bodies differently than we did when we were younger.

Now that I'm a parent, my community has further segmented into queers with kids and queers without kids. Parenting has reshaped the rhythms and temporality of my life in big and small ways, and I love how being with my kid invites me into a deep presence that feels outside "normal" time. Like queerness, being around children bends time. Things move both quickly and slowly; life is very structured and always fluid. I observe who in my circle knows how to move with that different rhythm and pace and who doesn't. It's made my circle smaller, a contraction that seems to go against the radical, community-oriented values we espouse. I feel alternately sad and mad about this, and disappointed. Why don't we know how to be with each other?

I notice parallels with how disabled people describe their experiences with the liberatory and challenging aspects of living inside of "crip time."[253] JD Davids, a chronically ill and intermittently disabled transmasculine person, describes himself as an "illder," an identity that has to do with "being an elder maybe faster than I would've been otherwise, who has learned some things by living with chronic illness."[254] Queer and trans disabled people share stories of isolation, too, not because disability is inherently isolating but because ableism creates the conditions for isolation, everything from stairs and inaccessible buildings to hours spent on the phone with social services to nondisabled people saying, "Your body is depressing."

There is a pattern here: A community broadly united under a common LGBTQ+ identity, yet divided along the lines of age, ability, and the degree to which we are dependent on other people or other people are dependent on us. There is loss in these divisions: loss of potential, pleasure, joy, and brilliance; loss of the wisdom and richness that comes with being part of a diverse and inclusive community; loss of survival strategies and mutual aid; loss of life.

In articulating a desire for greater interdependence, I'm mindful of how capitalism, colonialism, white supremacy, ableism, violence, and trauma have shaped my experiences of family and kinship, and how they've severed me from a more complex web of relations. I understand (in the limited ways my social locations enable me to) that in many contexts—particularly among Black, Indigenous, and people of colour and disabled people—interdependent, intergenerational communities are the norm, or they were before the violences of capitalism, colonialism, ableism, and white supremacy were enacted upon them. It feels important to acknowledge that I'm not articulating a radical vision for some new form of community. I'm dreaming of something different than what I'm able to perceive around me, something other people and communities already know how to do and have been doing for generations.

What will we need to re-learn, unlearn, or let go of to become more interdependent? For many of us, myself included, this will involve mentally and materially disentangling ourselves from the ways capitalism, colonialism, ableism, and white supremacy have shaped our perceptions of aging. It will mean cultivating an embodied practice of interdependence, redistributing resources, and learning how to be with each other's body/minds as they shift and change over time. It will mean believing that it's possible for more of us to get old, and that there are more ways to get old than we've been allowed or have allowed ourselves to imagine.

LIFE EXPECTANCY, OR WHY I WANT US TO EXPECT MORE LIFE AND FEEL ENTITLED TO IT

Getting older is complicated for us because queer and trans folks don't always expect to live, let alone live long enough to get old. People around us die young, often preventably and violently. We internalize messages that tell us we're at higher risk of sickness and death, that we're more likely to die than other people. For many people, the trauma, violence, and oppression we and our loved ones face translates into the sense of a shortened life expectancy, a belief in the inevitability that we will die sooner than others.

For example, trans women are often told their average life expectancy is thirty-five, a number I've heard trans women both younger and older than thirty-five repeat as if it's both true and inevitable. LGBTQ+ nonprofits quote it in their advocacy campaigns; celebrities cite it during awards shows. But a closer look shows this oft-cited number isn't grounded in reliable data.[255] I say this not to challenge the reality of the many forms of violence trans women face, or to deny the impact it has on their lives, but rather to ask us to think about what it does to a person when we keep telling them they're going to die by thirty-five.

This brings me to the idea of "life expectancy." Whose expectations are we talking about, anyway? Here I'm less interested in what statistics can tell us about how long different LGBTQ+ people might expect to live—though this information is salient here, because of what it reveals about the inequitable distribution of life chances within our communities—than I am in how long individual queer and trans people expect to live. How much living does society expect of us, and how does that translate into the messages we receive about the risks associated with our very existence and the potential length of our lives? How does it shape the assumptions that inform health care delivery or resource allocation? How does it shape our perceptions of ourselves and the possibility that we might have a future to look forward to?

How much life do we expect for ourselves or assume we're entitled to?

I recently went to a friend's birthday party. He's a trans man who was turning forty, and when I asked how he was feeling about celebrating his birthday, he expressed surprise and gratitude for having made it this far. I was struck by this sentiment, not because it was unusual but because it was so familiar. I'd heard it from other LGBTQ+ people before. Maybe some of you also feel surprised and glad you're still here. I'm glad you're still here. There's a lot standing in the way of queer and trans people's survival and making it one more day, one more year, sometimes even one more hour or minute, is a big deal. But I wish it didn't have to be.

I wish we lived in a world where we weren't constantly being told our lives were going to kill us and where more of us (all of us!) were able to live to old age. I want us to believe that we're going to get old, to look forward to it, to see it as a privilege and not something to be afraid of.

I want us to expect more life and feel entitled to it.

OLD, QUEER, AND THRIVING: SEEING
A LIFE FOR OURSELVES THROUGH TIME

If we're going to learn how to look forward to aging and believe it's possible to be old, queer, and thriving, we need examples and role models. We often think of this search in relation to the coming-out process, the idea that as young people we look for LGBTQ+ adults in our communities and in popular culture to help us figure out who we might be able to grow into. In reality, I think this search continues throughout our lives as queer and trans people.

Part of finding ourselves involves looking to others, often people older than us, for visions of how to live into the lives, relationships, and bodies we imagine for ourselves as we move through different stages of our lives: What can a queer parent look like? What is it like to be a middle-aged trans woman? How do disabled femme grandparents dress when they're cruising for dates? As we get older, it can be hard to find examples and role models because of how ageism and ableism serve to isolate older people in our communities, and because far too many of our peers and predecessors die before they have the opportunity to get old. Who will be our teachers in a community with too many beloved dead and too few elders?

In an interview, seventy-two-year-old writer, filmmaker, and activist Amber L. Hollibaugh describes the loneliness of not having older femmes in her life to look to as she ages:

> I do not have women older than myself to talk with about what aging does to an erotic identity. I don't have anybody that can say to me, "Oh, I remember when I was seventy-two, this started to happen. I remember when the first time my lover was really in a wheelchair and she was going to have to stay there, how we had to negotiate desire" ... I never saw a woman older than myself who was femme identified and queer ... that's a really lonely road. [256]

She continues, "I needed to always to see that there was a life for me through time, that I could live and be who I was erotically, be who I was sexually and ... politically." Hollibaugh connects this to her commitment to fostering relationships with and being a role model for femmes younger than her.

Yet these intergenerational dynamics aren't without their challenges as younger queer and trans people look around them for examples of what aging can look like. In an essay on aging, queer writer and educator Rose Cullis, who's in her sixties, shares a story of younger woman coming up to her after a performance and exclaiming, "I want to be just like you in twenty years!" Cullis writes, "I knew [she] meant well, but I wanted, somehow, to just be who I am and not some example of aging to strive for."[257] At the same time, she acknowledges the importance of mentorship and the power of seeing people older than us who embody aging in ways that feed our queer desires. We need proof that our futures are possible, that it's possible for us to be old, queer, and thriving.

I think this is the reason I've seen so many people share photos on social media from Jess T. Dugan and Vanessa Fabbre's portrait series of trans elders, *To Survive on This Shore*.[258] The portraits are glorious: image after image of trans people in their fifties, sixties, seventies, eighties, and nineties. Some are mundane shots of people dressed casually at home, others are more glamorous, my femme gaze drawn to the elders dressed in animal print, polka dots, faux fur, lace, and bright red feathers. I feel joy when I see tattooed, bearded bears holding each other; when I look at Miss Major's spiked leather cuff, leopard-print cane, and take-no-bullshit expression; when I notice the pleasure on a trans man's face as he sits in his wheelchair and his partner kisses him on the forehead. Some people smile in their portraits; others gaze steadily at the camera. I see a strength and a kind of defiance in all of their faces and it's beautiful.

These portraits feed a deep hunger for tangible examples of what aging can look like. When my friends shared them on social media, I felt a sense of relief in their posts, a kind of whole-body exhale that comes along with seeing concrete proof of something—someone—you needed to know existed because it means you might be able to exist like that, too. We need to know that getting older doesn't have to mean becoming someone different or making ourselves smaller or less vibrant.

BEYOND RAINBOW NURSING HOMES

While doing research for this essay, I noticed that a lot of the literature on LGBTQ+ aging focuses on how to make nursing homes and long-term care facilities more welcoming and inclusive to queer and trans folks. I understand why this work is necessary in a context where people may have fewer family members to care for them in a way that enables them to age in place, and where the provision of home care is woefully inadequate to meet the needs of people living in the community. I also understand that for some people, like those who have complex health needs that require 24/7 access to specialized equipment and support or who don't want to age and die at home, having access to full-time care in an institutional context may feel like their best or only option.

Still, this focus on LGBTQ+-affirming nursing homes feels like a failure of imagination to me, like we're not dreaming far enough into what's possible. The idea of living in institutional environments like long-term care evokes considerable fear and anxiety among LGBTQ+ older adults. Research has documented their concerns about experiencing discrimination from staff or other residents, being separated from partners and cut off from chosen family, or having to go back into the closet in order to live safely.[259] Trans and gender-diverse older adults fear they will experience transphobic violence from staff and other residents in long-term care.[260] They express concerns about being outed, being denied care, or not being able to express their gender identities. Bisexual older adults, who experience biphobia, stigma, and lack of social support, may experience further marginalization in these facilities.[261] LGBTQ+ older adults who are Indigenous, Black, and people of colour may also experience racism from facility staff and/or other residents. Indigenous older adults, many of whom already experience housing insecurity and/or overcrowding driven by chronic underfunding and colonial government (in)action, lack access to culturally safe housing that meets their needs.

COVID-19's massive death toll among residents and staff in long-term care facilities drew attention to how living and working inside these carceral spaces contributes to and causes death. These deaths are disproportionately experienced by older adults, disabled people, and the people who care for them, the majority of whom are women of colour. COVID-19's horrifying impact on the long-term care sector is amplifying calls for abolition of these facilities, especially from disabled activists. I'm paying attention to those calls, and that's why my dreams of a world without carceral institutions includes the abolition of the current model of long-term care. I want us to embody and practise the idea that no one is "too much" to have their needs met in community. As queer disabled attorney and activist Katie Tastrom reminds us, "Abolition is as much about building the appropriate resources and supports as it is about tearing down the harmful structures that cage, torture, and kill us."[262]

In saying this, it's important to acknowledge the long history of activism by disabled people (including many who are queer and trans) to end institutionalization, stay out of nursing homes, and increase access to community supports. An example of this is the 1999 *Olmstead* decision, in which two disabled women, Lois Curtis and Elaine Wilson, successfully sued the US government for access to community-based services after spending years waiting to leave an institution due to lack of access to services in the community.[263] More recently, disabled people in the United States have been fighting cuts to Medicaid, a program that provides health coverage to millions of people in the United States. These cuts would eliminate many disabled people's ability to live in their homes with the support of publicly funded attendants who assist them with personal care.[264] In Canada, disabled activist and advocate Jonathan Marchand, who lives in a Quebec long-term care facility, spent five nights in a cage outside the provincial legislature in August 2020 during the COVID-19 pandemic. He was protesting the dangerous living conditions in these facilities and lack of access to the supports disabled and older people need to remain in their communities.[265]

Older people are also advocating for change and dreaming new possibilities into being. In France, Thérèse Clerc spent thirteen years working with fellow feminist activists, all older women, to lobby the government to build a self-managed residence called Baba Yaga House. The six-storey apartment building opened in 2012; it has twenty-five apartments and includes a large ground-floor space that serves as an open university for the local community where residents run courses, give concerts, do creative writing, and offer discussion groups.[266] A group of women in Toronto were so inspired by this French example that they're working to organize something similar there.[267] There's also Roze Hallen, a cooperative "living-apart-together" community in Amsterdam created in 2014 by nineteen LGBTQ+ older adults who wanted to grow old together. Four years later, residents moved into the fourteen-unit building, where they each have their own apartment, along with an extra one for when they need a paid caregiver like a nurse or home care worker to stay there, too.

There's Carefree Boulevard, a resort and RV park in Fort Meyers, Florida, that's home to over 500 women between the ages of forty and eighty-five, most of them lesbians. It's got a dance floor, a lake to kayak in, a library, and a kiln, among other amenities. An article about the community quotes one resident as saying, "I have never felt so free in any place I have lived, in my seventy-five years." Another said, "I love going to the dances here. It has become my 'bar' scene of my earlier days."[268]

In searching for possibilities, I also look to the stories of individual elders, like Miss Major, now in her eighties, creating House of GG (a.k.a. the Griffin-Gracy Educational Retreat and Historical Center) in Little Rock, Arkansas. Multidisciplinary artist, great-grandmother, and self-described "transformed woman who loves women" Aiyyana Maracle spent the last six years of her life at home on the Six Nations Reservation, where she died surrounded by loving family and friends. Lesbian activist Phyllis Lyon, who had dementia, was able to live in her own home until she died at age ninety-five thanks to the help of a group of paid queer and trans caregivers organized by Lyon's daughter, Kendra Mon, a social worker, and Lyon's friend and long-time bookkeeper, Pan Haskins. This team of caregivers was funded by Lyon's friends, mostly wealthy older lesbians, who will be repaid when Lyon's house is sold.[269] There's also disabled Puerto Rican Jewish writer and activist Aurora Levins Morales, now in her mid-sixties. She's part of a movement she's calling rematriation, "the return, in particular, of middle aged and old women, loaded with skills, dreams and purpose, to become part of the enriched soil of resistance of Puerto Rico."[270] After finding herself homeless in the United States as a result of environmental illness, she built The Vehicle for Change, a chemically accessible and partially sustainable home on wheels that now sits on Finca La Lluvia, her family's land in Puerto Rico.[271]

I'm intrigued by all of these examples, and they also raise questions for me, like what are the limitations of a self-managed or detached home–style model for people with more significant access or care needs? And what about all the LGBTQ+ people living in poverty who can't afford to buy a house or buy their way into a community? What does it look like to create age-friendly communities for LGBTQ+ people in ways that honour Indigenous sovereignty and stewardship of the land? I don't have the answers to these questions, but it's critical we engage with them as we imagine different possibilities for the futures of queer and trans aging.

I'M NOT GETTING ANY YOUNGER AND NEITHER ARE YOU: NOW WHAT?

If you know anything about eldercare today, you know there's a big gap between my dreams and our reality (hence: my nightmares). To realize the kinds of changes I describe in this essay will require systemic transformation, which is admittedly my jam, even if it may not be achievable in my lifetime. But I'm not getting any younger and neither are you, so what should we do now? Well, for one thing I'd like us to begin imagining the possibility of getting old and figuring out what would help us welcome that possibility. Just because you don't consider yourself old now doesn't mean you can't begin to plan for life as you age.

Talk about your hopes, dreams, and practical stuff with the close people in your life. If possible, get the necessary paperwork and documentation in place to ensure that those people understand your wants and needs around things like end-of-life care and are empowered to make decisions on your behalf if they need to. I know that this kind of paperwork can feel alienating and overwhelming to folks for all kinds of reasons, and it can be expensive and hard to find queer- and trans-affirming experts to help with the more technical stuff. I'd love to see the creation of collectives that provide community members with accessible, sliding-scale legal, logistical, and emotional support around navigating their own care and end-of-life planning.

I also want us to begin fostering more intergenerational, interdependent communities. I feel curious about the kinds of possibilities we could create through accessible, intergenerational cohousing or cooperative housing communities in urban and rural contexts where people of different ages and abilities could live together. In my imagined community, there'd be a playground and a daycare for kids, a community garden, and gathering spaces for people to cook, create, practise their faiths, organize, have fun, and spend time together. There'd be lots of private spaces, too, so folks can enjoy whatever degrees of solitude makes them happiest (introverts get old, too!). The community would have a range of styles of living spaces accessible to people with different bodies and health needs, as well as free or affordable access to whatever home care, professional health supports, and other services people need to thrive. Paid caregivers would be compensated generously and treated with respect, and unpaid caregivers would feel well-supported to care for their loved ones in ways that feel sustainable to them.

If you're currently housed, you can do an accessibility audit of your home or apartment building and look for opportunities to make it more accessible now or in the near future, for you or anyone else who needs it. If you're younger or at mid-life, is there a way you can build relationships with and be of service to elders in your community? If yes, figure out how and do it. Not sure where to find them? Reach out to your local LGBTQ+ organization or national organizations like Canada's Senior Pride Network or US-based SAGE: Advocacy and Services for LGBT Elders. Look to examples like the mentorship program at Kofi House, a Detroit-based community space for lesbian and queer women and girls that pairs youth with older lesbian mentors to pass on their stories and histories.[272]

If you have the capacity, look for ways to begin organizing at the level of your local community, including supporting LGBTQ+ older adults who are isolated to develop networks of chosen family and support. Advocate for increased access to free and affordable paid care and better working conditions for caregivers. And if you have any sort of decision-making authority over LGBTQ+ older adults' lives, for goodness' sake please think beyond rainbow nursing homes. We deserve more and better than that.

I have dreams and nightmares about aging as a queer person, and I oscillate between hope and fear about getting old. I still want to get old, though—really, *really* old—and I want you to get really, *really* old, too. I want to see your beautiful, wrinkled faces, your white hair, your bent bodies, your canes and mobility devices. I want to see the ways time and experience accumulate on our bodies, how we'll look at fifty, sixty, seventy, eighty, ninety, maybe even a hundred. I want our great-grandchildren to live in a community where they're surrounded by queer and trans elders who can show them a world of possibilities for how to be and who they might be through time. May their hunger for possibilities always be satiated and may ours be, too.

The Emancipatory Potential of Aging

Interview with Hannah Kia

Hannah Kia, PhD, RCSW, is an assistant professor at the University of British Columbia's School of Social Work in Vancouver, BC. Her research centres on LGBTQ/2+ aging and health, a program of study that draws on Hannah's lived experiences as a trans woman and queer person and growing up as a newcomer in Canada. Before becoming an academic, Hannah practised as a social worker in acute care and hospice palliative care. Our conversation weaves these themes together as we explore the emancipatory potential of aging and the complexities of LGBTQ/2+ aging in a context of neoliberalism.

Zena: What drew you to study aging?

Hannah: I came of age when the height of the HIV/AIDS epidemic was really abating. I have vivid memories from my childhood of adults telling me things like, "I really hope you're not queer because if you are, you're going to grow old alone and without a family. That's going to be your fate." The language of fate was very central to these oppressive narratives. As a queer person who was also a newcomer to Canada, I wasn't being exposed to other queer people or culture very much during this time, so I didn't have a sense of alternative possibilities.

 As an adult, I became a social worker. I started my social work practice in an urban hospital where my colleagues were queer positive, though at the time conversations about being trans positive weren't happening very openly. While my colleagues were well-intentioned, the system was constructed in such a way that whenever I encountered queer and trans people accessing health care in my capacity as a social worker, I would notice that their issues, needs, and experiences were, on the one hand, either ignored or rendered invisible or, on the other hand, responded to completely inappropriately.

I noticed that a lot of folks accessing services would often be left in situations of great vulnerability without any kind of appropriate supports in place to mitigate the issues accompanying the vulnerabilities they faced as a result of these systemic failures. So that's where my passion for aging research, specifically in relation to queer and trans lives, took root. I wanted to learn more about how queer and trans people cared for one another as they aged, both the rich, beautiful stories and the more difficult ones that reflect the influence of oppressive forces on our lives.

Zena: What are some of the things you've observed about the queer and trans community's attitudes and perspectives on aging?

Hannah: Part of the beauty of queer and trans lives is the diversity of our experiences, which shows up in our experiences of aging. There are tremendous generational differences in how folks relate to queer and trans identities and what that means for them in terms of whether they want that dimension of their identity to be seen, and to what extent, as they age.

Some queer and trans folks consider it necessary to express their queerness or transness in the context of aging. Others want these aspects of their identities to be a more private or intimate aspect of their lives. Both are perfectly valid choices. I think these differences are something we need to think about more in relation to the varied ways people make sense of and experience aging, and what kinds of services and supports they might need as a result.

I also think queer and trans people have unique issues in the context of aging. On the one hand, queer and trans people may have rich families of choice, but on the other hand, some of us may lack access to our families of origin. We live in a context of neoliberalism that has privatized and limited access to care, and often rests on the assumption that people will be able to rely on their spouse or families of origin to care for them as we age. There are so many queer and trans folks who, as a result of lacking access to their families of origin and the supports they need to continue living in the community, end up being coerced into situations where they transition into residential care environments. And that can be a very scary prospect for a lot of queer and trans people.

Zena: In your writing you've explored the idea of hypervisibility in relation to the more common narrative of LGBTQ+ people becoming invisible as we age. Tell me more about this and what it means in terms of the well-being of queer and trans older adults.

Hannah: A lot of the research and writing on LGBTQ+ aging focuses on the invisibility and erasure of older queer and trans lives. The silencing of older queer and trans lives and a shortage of research on aging in our communities can lead to professions like nursing, social work, rehabilitation sciences, and others not being informed about the unique experiences and needs of older queer and trans adults. You end up with a whole health care system that is then developed without accounting for the issues of older LGBTQ+ people.

While it's true that queer and trans aging is invisible in many contexts, I argue there are ways we also become hypervisible as we age. Neoliberal ideology favours the individual, the nuclear family, and normative family structures and relationships. If you conform to this norm, you're less visible to and less at risk of being disciplined or controlled by the state. Queer and trans family structures come under far greater scrutiny than those of people who live in hetero-, cis-, mono-, and amatonormative family structures. We are punished for existing in contexts of interdependence that are validating to our identities, because these come under scrutiny a lot more than normative family structures do.

For example, we may be more likely to be coerced into residential care facilities as we age, because home care providers might assume we don't have kin-based caregivers and are therefore incapable of successfully aging at home in our communities (sometimes referred to as "aging in place") without these normative family structures.

When and if we end up in settings like residential care facilities, we may end up labelled as LGBTQ+—sometimes without our consent—and then face the repercussions of being intelligibly "different" (or hypervisible) within these dominant systems. For example, a woman in a residential care facility who is visited by a seemingly same-gender partner might, without her consent, be labelled a "lesbian" by residents and care staff. Because of this, she might be targeted with violence, harassment, and discrimination at the facility since these kinds of state institutions are often not set up to support care recipients—as well as unpaid caregivers—existing outside of a normative family structure.

Zena: I'm interested in the idea that queerness and transness bend time, in the sense that we simultaneously stay young for longer and get older sooner. Does this idea resonate with you? How does it layer onto your reflections about caring relationships among trans folks and transfeminine people in particular?

Hannah: We have the idea of staying young cohabiting with the idea of aging prematurely. I think these two ideas exist in tension in queer and trans communities. The reason we're challenged in terms of being able to place them in a linear way is because our whole thinking around aging has been shaped by a very cisnormative, heteronormative model of the life course—the idea that you're born, you grow up, you fall in love, you get married, you have kids, your kids grow up, you get old, and then you die.

When it comes to transfeminine people, part of where I struggle with notions of aging is that there's still this dominant narrative around not only aging prematurely but also having a lower life expectancy. We end up being elders for one another in ways that wouldn't make sense to people who are not queer and even some people who are queer but aren't trans.

I remember being in a conversation with a transfeminine person who was five years younger than me. To her, I was an elder and this felt very flattering to me. It also felt tragic because I so badly wanted this young person to have what I would imagine to be a "true" elder in her life. I really felt like I was still not far enough into my own life to be able to offer her what she was searching for. Yet we are in positions where we have to provide one another with that kind of caring labour because we simply don't have the mothers, fathers, or parents that are available to people who are cis or people who are non-queer.

It's interesting how this dynamic ends up working. It creates beautiful opportunities for reshaping and challenging the confines of normative conceptualizations of the life course. It also reflects the very difficult realities that a lot of trans people have to live with. In particular, the violence that ends up cutting a lot of our lives short.

Zena: I've been writing about life expectancy and my observation that so many queer and trans people are surprised they're still alive.

Hannah: That's definitely a reality for trans and queer people. I certainly had an awareness of my trans identity from a very young age. But I ruled out transition until I was thirty. I adopted a queer identity for much of my childhood, adolescence, and adulthood until I started transitioning, even though I did this privately during my younger years. Because of the messages I'd received growing up about many queer people only living until their twenties and thirties during the height of HIV/AIDS epidemic, I didn't expect to live beyond thirty, so I built a life narrative for myself that didn't really take into account what aging would look like.

I think a lot of queer and trans folks are in this predicament. I've been privileged enough to have the opportunity to live authentically. And yet, I still have this amount of life left and what do I do with it, and how do I make it meaningful? These are questions I ask myself and that I see reflected in the stories I hear from my research participants—questions around meaning and family as we enter middle adulthood and later stages of our lives.

Zena: It makes me think of something you wrote in a paper looking at the experiences of older gay men. In it, you talked about the emancipatory potential of these older queer bodies. I would love to hear you talk more about what that means to you, what you learned about it in the context of your research, and how you think it might have the potential to disrupt common stereotypes or narratives about aging as a queer or a trans person.

Hannah: A lot of the gay men in one of my studies would talk about how, when they would enter health care settings, they would make themselves identifiable as HIV-positive. Their HIV status would be synonymous with queerness in a lot of those settings, even though we've gone through generations of trying to disentangle gay men from the HIV epidemic. In relation to this idea of visibility, HIV is something that outs people as having a queer body, a body that is non-normative in some way.

Some of the men who participated in my study really took pride in being positive. They saw opportunities in laying claim to their positive bodies and using their bodies to educate providers, and in that way working toward systems change. I remember one of my research participants talking passionately about how, although he had been heavily marginalized in mainstream health settings as a result of being gay and HIV-positive, he joined community groups mandated with advocating for better patient conditions and had capitalized on those opportunities to make his voice heard as an HIV-positive person. In this way, he used his body to cultivate change.

Zena: If you could offer advice to queer and trans older adults on how to advocate for themselves in the health system, what would it be?

Hannah: I see emancipatory potential in making ourselves visible in health care contexts, in other institutional contexts where our voices might be silenced or used against us, grounded in careful reflection on our social positions and whether there are specific spaces where we might feel safe to make ourselves visible.

On the one hand, there are, for example, trans folks who have gone on to "live stealth" because they needed to. They do not disclose that they're trans, they do not make themselves visible, and that is a perfectly valid decision because it usually comes from a place of careful reflection on whether the spaces they're in are safe for them to be visible or not.

On the other hand, queer and trans folks who are in relative positions of power and advantage need to practise finding spaces where we can make ourselves visible and have our voices heard, because I think that's a place where we can begin a process of cultivating change. For trans people like me who are in relative positions of power and privilege, this presents opportunities for us to use our bodies to draw attention to the idea that what's often seen as "non-normative" is just a variation on the body as it ages. I'm really excited at the prospect of aging and being able to use my body in this way.

I'm approaching this with a little bit of trepidation because, already, my experiences with health care systems haven't always been the greatest. That being said, I have a lot of hope and I think we have to start by making ourselves visible. That's what I mean by "emancipatory potential," making ourselves visible to hopefully work toward a better world for queer and trans folks who are aging.

Zena: If you could offer health care providers who are caring for queer and trans older adults advice on how to provide more liberatory care, what would it be?

Hannah: Honour control and autonomy. Starting from there is absolutely critical because there are so many variations on what being queer and trans actually means to folks as we age, how we relate to those identities, and whether or not we want people around us to know we identify in these ways. Health care systems and health care providers are responsible for creating conditions that allow queer and trans older adults to have full control and choice over how we make ourselves visible, if at all, in health care systems. Every other practice should stem from this starting point.

For example, follow older adults' lead in terms of language use and pronoun use, even if it's sometimes counterintuitive. When I was practising as a social worker, one of my patients was a gay man who identified as gender nonconforming and used "he" pronouns. A lot of well-meaning practitioners at my place of work started referring to him as "she" and "her." This was profoundly stigmatizing for this person and outed him as being gender nonconforming; he then became a target of violence from other patients.

Zena: It often seems to me like the queer and trans community is very age segmented. Does that resonate for you? How can we build more intergenerational, age-friendly, and interdependent LGBTQ+ communities?

Hannah: It definitely resonates with me. I'm fortunate to have relationships with some older queer and trans folks who I very much see as mentors and as wonderful family of choice for me. And yet I often feel like there are so many folks out there who I could learn from and there would be no way for me to find them. I suspect there are a lot of people in my age category who are longing for connection across generations and struggle to find it. I think what this points to is the need for a greater number and quality of structures that allow for cross-generational connections in queer and trans communities.

There are local organizations that have started programs providing peer-to-peer connections between younger and older folks who are queer and trans. I'd like to see us create more room for programs like this in the health system—for example, a peer navigation program for older queer and trans folks who are navigating health care systems, being paired with somebody who also identifies as queer and trans and might have some experience as a service provider as well. We also need to create peer-run programs in community organizations where cross-generational connections are really the main point of those programs and where there's a lead person connecting people across generations.

Zena: It makes me think of examples like cohousing communities where people live in closely clustered private homes or apartments and share common spaces like big community kitchens, play areas for children, et cetera. What would it look like to live in a way where there was more age mixing and more mixing of the different skills, knowledge, and ways of caring for one another that we each bring to the table?

Hannah: I think cohousing is a beautiful idea and I think we need to really be transparent about the neoliberal regime we're in right now. We need to push bureaucracies at all levels of government to actually support cohousing arrangements. Because sometimes in the professionalized health literature, cohousing is presented as an opportunity for families to "achieve independence" from the state, meaning families are left to fend for themselves—essentially, that because these cohoused families exist, the state is absolved of any responsibility.

Ideally, we need cohousing or other similar living arrangements that are supported by the state. So, you know, you have people who are aging in place not only being supported by kin-based and other informal caregivers and offering something in return to these caregivers, but you also have a state-sanctioned role for services that are meant to support those caregivers in doing the work they're doing.

I recently lost my own mother. She had a stroke several years ago and after her stroke, she continued being one of the most brilliant, wonderful people I've ever known in my life, just an amazing person. I was one of my mother's caregivers, along with other family members. My mother, our family, and I would have loved for her to stay at home with us, but we didn't have the support necessary to make this possible. My mom needed two people to be present with her round the clock because she needed skilled care to do everyday activities like get out of bed.

If we'd had access to skilled nursing care in our home, it would have allowed us to help my mother age in place for the last few years of her life. It would have very much been a reciprocal arrangement, because our relationship was such an important source of love and care for me, and if my mother had been able to stay at home with us, she would have been able to care for me as well.

Unfortunately, that's not what happened because we are in a period of austerity that limits people's access to care. So yes to cohousing and other ways of living together in intergenerational communities, *and* we need much greater access to caregiving and other supports provided by state structures in non-invasive ways. All these supports should be rooted in respect for people's dignity, control, and autonomy and honour their identities and the important relationships in their lives.

Libera me

Joshua Wales

Even from a distance, I can tell you're looking for someone. The porter pushes your stretcher down the white hallway to your new room. Your eyes dart from face to face: nurses, social workers, volunteers. You only smile at some of them.

Your stretcher passes me as I write notes at the nursing station. Your hair is thick grey waves, but your cheeks have been hollowed out. You seize on something—you smile as if we're old friends. It takes up your whole face. I'm not wearing floral, my hair is symmetrical, I'm holding myself in my usual stillness, hands safely occupied with pen and paper. But even so, you see me, or through me, and I see you, and our mutual nods feel like an exhalation. This is how we start.

Your main source of discomfort, you tell me, is the banal colour scheme of this palliative care unit. The off-cream walls with beige trim. The worn terrazzo floors. You squint at my dress shirt, ivory with a pattern of light blue squares only visible from up close. Even the winter sunlight, reflected off the glass and steel buildings that rise around us, is pale. You almost miss the grotesque crucifixes affixed to every wall of the Catholic hospital that transferred you here, after refusing to provide medical assistance in dying. "Sure, those folks may deprive you of your human rights, but by God, they know how to create some visual drama!"

I sit in the chair beside you. Folded in my lap is the paperwork, just in case you want to get the process started. They are multipage checklists, litanies of suffering. Certification of your right to die. I can already tell your answers won't fit in the boxes.

But it's been a long day. You're exhausted. When you cough, the rims of your eyes redden. You're not in any rush to die, you say. You want a few days, or a few weeks, to talk it out with me. You're suddenly worried about dying in a place like this—an institutional box, a perfect square, all right angles.

Sitting up in bed, you hold an imaginary cigarette to your lips, inhaling deeply. When you exhale, you release the invisible smoke rings in my direction. The square of light from the window doesn't reach your bed.

"Doc, do you have any bad habits?" you ask.

"I guess I spend too much time on my phone?"

"They told me I got this cancer because of my bad habits. I've got *many* bad habits." You list these off on your fingers. "Smoking, fisting, blasphemy, violent protesting, swearing, double denim, slashing the tires of white supremacists, spitting, insisting on spending holidays with my family." You cough. "That last one is the only one I wouldn't recommend, by the way."

One day, you tell me about yelling therapy. You went to a therapist who told you that if you just yelled loud enough, it would cure your anxiety.

"Who did you yell at?" I ask.

"The old white straight man living rent-free in the back of my mind. I could never see his face. Didn't know who he was. But his arms were always folded, just watching. Making sure I moved, thought, wrote, spoke, sang, dressed—just the way he wanted." You wonder if I have someone like this living in the back of my mind as well.

I don't answer right away, and you add: "Medicine must always be trying to fold you down into its box, dulling you, painting you with one colour." You grab the turquoise plastic basin beside you, cough, spit out blood-streaked sputum.

I race to push aside all the dusty furniture piled in the back of my head. And there he is. I can't see his face clearly. His arms are folded. I'm startled to find him there, but I'm not surprised.

I tried to choose a better shirt today: navy, but with a checkered pattern. You're unconvinced.

The social worker visits you to offer spiritual care. I don't have to work hard to eavesdrop because your voice, hoarse as it is, can be heard down the hallway.

You kindly decline her service but thank her for coming. You ask her to send in the Hospital Fag instead. "You know," you say as if you're trying to jog her memory, "the Official Hospital Fag, the one who wears a bedazzled name tag and leather sash, and comes to talk to me about how they make this space, you know, super queer for me. How they can accommodate my specific shades of queerness. Make sure all my queer needs are met? You—you guys don't have one?"

Today you don't want to talk about your own death. My daily check-ins, all the questions about yourself, are tiring. Instead, you want to tell me about the deaths of your friends, who have died in many different ways, of many different things. Today, we spend a lot of time sitting in silence.

I check in to see how the weekend went. You say you like my new shirt—"Purple diagonal stripes, getting bolder!"—and you complain that the hospital's ice chips are too small, and tell me the pain in your chest is getting stronger.

But there's more. My colleague saw you over the weekend. He walked in like he had no time. He kept getting your name wrong, kept using a name that was not part of you. And when you corrected, he smirked and non-apologized, and this felt like a kind of violence. You fired him on the spot, told him you did not need a weekend doctor.

"You know, before, when I'd go to the hospital, I tried to un-queer myself. It was like pouring litres of matte beige paint all over my body—it settled on my vocal cords, weighed down my limbs, suffocated my skin. But I kept pouring because I was afraid of what a straight doctor would say about me to their colleagues. Or what the nurse would think about my *lifestyle*. And whether—deep down, in their most honest place—they would think I was worthy of their care."

I leave the room to call that colleague. I intend it to be a flamboyantly, carelessly, ferociously angry phone call, a phone call that will crack the walls, peel the paint off. But he tells me I'm overreacting, I've misunderstood, I should calm down and, to my eternal shame, I do: I lower my voice, remove my expletives; I don't cry. I haven't found the cure for the man in the back of my head.

Once, we laugh so loudly that a nurse comes to shut the door, tells us to keep it down.

The light in your room is late-afternoon yellow. Your eyes are redder, your voice hoarser. You say you can feel yourself disappearing, like a stamp running out of ink. I move my chair closer so you can speak more quietly.

You cough, then spit into your basin. I rest my elbows on the pink-and-grey blanket that a friend has knitted for you. Your eyes squint shut with effort, as the muscles of your chest strain against their own resistance.

You lean your head back to rest against the pillow. To look directly at your death, you tell me, is to look straight into the sun. Painful. There is the instinct to look away, to seek the shade. But if you keep your gaze there for a few extra seconds, spots of light begin to dance in your eyes like fireworks. Like a celebration. You're ready to be cele-brated. You're ready to finish off the paperwork, to set a date.

As I get up to leave, you stop me and say, with the sobriety of a deathbed confession: "I want to die with someone sitting on my face."

"I'll see what I can do," I say, with equal solemnity.

You close your eyes and smile. "What, so all of a sudden nothing can shock you?"

On the day you die, I enter your room carrying a tray of vials. One of the vials is full of propofol; seeing its thick, viscous whiteness, you say, wryly, "What the *fuck* are you injecting me with?"

You tell me you like my mesh shirt.

There are a dozen people gathered around you, and you explain to me that each one of them has dated at least two others in the room. Someone is reading Tarot in the corner. Another is yarn-bombing your hospital bed. Another has brought an autoharp and is playing Tracy Chapman and k.d lang.

There's incense burning, and someone is waving the smoke away from the smoke detector. There's a bowl of clip-on nose rings, a selection of herbal teas, a bowl of MDMA, a box of dress-up clothes, a karaoke machine (but that is for after, you say). There's no dancing because you always hated dancing, hated feeling hot and claustro-phobic, hated loud noises.

Everyone is wearing a strap-on of various shades, shapes, and sizes; they droop in deference, a sign of respect, you tell me. Someone does offer to sit on your face, but you laugh and tell them you're not actually in the mood.

At your request, someone turns on the "Libera me" from Verdi's *Requiem* and it plays with a soft urgency before fading to nothing. Someone reads James Baldwin: "It seems to me that one ought to rejoice in the fact of death—ought to decide, indeed, to earn one's death by confronting with passion the conundrum of life."

You look around at us. No one's arms are folded. The backs of our minds belong only to ourselves.

As I begin to run the medications into your veins, there is a deep silence. Within it, I can almost hear the cracking open of the beige walls, the shatter of paint layers falling to the floor in pieces. The room feels unbound, as if the walls can finally breathe easily, flexible enough to hold your shape.

You start to drift off. You smile as your eyes close.

"I guess this is me."

Put Me in the Living Room and Cover Me with Flowers

Queering Death

Zena Sharman

The morning my mom died a nurse called from the hospital to tell me the news. I'd been expecting a call like this one, but it still shocked me when it happened. Moments before my phone rang, I was eating breakfast with my friends Jess, Amy, and their two young children in their kitchen. The room was cheerful and chaotic the way things are when you're dining with toddlers. It felt homey and almost normal, except for the part of me that had spent the past week anxiously wondering if my mother was going to die.

I left the warm conviviality of the kitchen table to take the call, already feeling numb. The nurse asked me to come to the hospital. I didn't understand why and assumed she needed me to sign some paperwork; somebody died, so I figured there had to be forms involved. I'd never lost a close family member before and I didn't know what to expect: I was a queer person in my mid-thirties, the only child of a single mother navigating through death's unfamiliar territory without a map to guide me.

I don't remember how I got to the hospital, though I assume Jess drove me. She and Amy had been offering me a home base for years every time I travelled back to Thunder Bay, the small northern city where I grew up, to care for my mom. Jess is a queer femme, like me, a naturopath with a background in supporting survivors of sexual assault, and Amy co-owns and cooks for a restaurant she founded with several other women. They care tangibly—rides to the airport; delicious, nourishing meals; clean sheets on the bed in their spare room; a few carefully placed acupuncture needles from Jess while I lay on their couch at the end of a long day. Their queer care steadied me during a time when I often felt like I was unravelling.

It wasn't the same hospital I went to when I was growing up. This one was newer, built after they shut down the two smaller local hospitals. Tall wooden columns jutted into the sky around the front of the rounded, modern-looking glass building. I entered the airy lobby through the main doors and found my way back to the ward where my mom had spent the past four days after a fall in her apartment contributed to a rapid decline in her health. There, a nurse in pastel scrubs ushered me into my mother's hospital room, where I was unprepared to be alone with her body. She'd been sick for six years and I knew she was going to die, but I wasn't ready to see her small, still frame under a blanket.

The night before, one of the hospital chaplains, an Indigenous man who remembered my mother from community gatherings, had led me and several of her closest friends and caregivers through a farewell ritual in her hospital room. The chaplain rested his eagle feather on the wool blanket we'd brought from home that was draped across my mom's legs. We took turns speaking to her about what she meant to us. She seemed peaceful in this moment, even though I knew her body was working hard to breathe.

The next morning, her hospital room felt too quiet, somehow both stifling and cavernous. I remember feeling conflicted as I stood at my mother's bedside. Part of me wanted to find sacredness and connection in that final moment with her. The other part of me wanted to get out of there as fast as possible because the experience felt like more than I was capable of holding alone. I stayed with her for a while, resting my hand on my mom's chest and talking to her, but I left quickly, carrying a bag of her things in my hand. Shame washed over me as I worried the nurse might think I was a bad daughter for leaving the room so soon.

It was the one time in my life I wanted so badly to be part of a religious community, to be rooted in a tradition and set of practices that would tell me what to do when someone dies. I wanted a community of older, wiser adults with shared values to swoop in and help me through the process: *This is how we wash the body; this is what we do with the body; this is how we say goodbye; this is how we mourn.* I wanted to be held and I wanted something to hold on to. I felt unmoored by death. I needed a sturdy container where I could let my grief run wild and I imagined that being part of a religious community might feel that way.

What I had instead was queerness, and the do-it-yourself (DIY) mindset I'd learned from the queer community. Queerness gave me the tools I needed to build my own container for the grief I felt losing my mom and eventually helped me find my way into a more healing relationship with death and dying.

Both my experience with my mom's death and my own work as an LGBTQ+ health advocate have me wondering what it would look like to queer death, and what queering death might offer the LGBTQ+ community as a means of individual and collective healing. What would have to change for us to die well, and for our loved ones to be held in their grief? How might creating or reclaiming our own personal and group rituals around death and dying help facilitate this change? How does all this fit into larger efforts to transform common beliefs and practices about death? And how is it connected to movements for racial, economic, and environmental justice?

DEATH, DIY QUEER STYLE

After my mom died, I felt like an orphan. My grief was an unruly, ever-shifting mix of emotions that would leave me unexpectedly crying on the bus, zoning out by binge-watching episodes of *Call the Midwife*, or channelling the overwhelmingness into frantically making spreadsheets to track the endless to-do lists that come with death. My experience growing up as a nonreligious white settler in Canada meant I'd unconsciously internalized a death-avoidant culture. We deny death, we don't talk about it, and we're only allowed to grieve if we follow an ableist, capitalist script: be sad, but not *too* sad; don't be *too much* or *too messy*; and get back to *normal* as quickly as possible so you can be productive again.

If I'd followed this limiting script, I wouldn't have been able to grieve in a way that felt authentic or healing to me. It's why I looked to queerness and the queer community for alternatives. They gave me the space and support I needed to be messy and weird in my grief, to make it up as I went along, to come undone and trust that someone would be there to help stitch me back together.

There's something inherently creative about being queer—that's why it's a noun *and* a verb. We're adept at the work of imagination, transformation, and creation. We defy norms and stereotypes throughout our lives as we make and remake our identities, families, and communities to reflect the visions we hold for ourselves and how we want to live. I brought this spirit into the experience of losing my mom. Since I didn't have a faith tradition or knowledge of my ancestral practices to guide me, I did something queer and trans people are so good at: I did it myself, with help from my friends and community.

The day she died, I gathered a group of my mother's close friends at dusk on the bank of a creek she held sacred, where we stood knee-deep in late-spring snow and laughed, cried, and shared our memories of her. In those raw early hours of my grief, it helped to be with other people who were also mourning my mom in a ritual of remembrance, something I'd first learned to do from other queer folks while mourning the deaths of LGBTQ+ people in our community.

Paying a funeral home to organize my mom's memorial felt too formal, not to mention expensive. I didn't trust that they would be queer-competent enough to work with me and I felt afraid of getting boxed into a staid traditional memorial that didn't reflect my mom's activist spirit. So, a couple of months later, I used the skills I'd developed from years of organizing and hosting queer dance parties and cabarets to help plan my mom's memorial service. I figured organizing and emceeing a memorial service wasn't all that different from the queer cabarets I'd organized before—except without the burlesque performers and drag queens.

Her memorial was in a Unitarian church we borrowed with help from Jess and Amy, who were members of the congregation. The space was bright and open with warm wooden pews and a place for kids to play. We covered a table near the front of the room in small objects and knick-knacks from my mom's apartment, kitschy figurines from the 1950s and 1960s mixed in with colourful wooden boxes and beautiful stones.

I invited people to choose a memento from the table, a suggestion from an older queer friend who'd already lost several family members and generously helped guide me through the logistics of death. It turned out to be a gesture both meaningful and practical. I'd spent the past week with my then-partner and my long-time friend Matt, a gay man who'd travelled 1,500 kilometres to help me. Together, we undertook the massive task of packing up my mom's apartment and distributing her many belongings to family, friends, and local charities. We needed homes for all that stuff.

The service itself was simple, just me and a few relatives and close friends sharing memories of my mom and speaking about our love for her and the impacts of her activism. Afterwards, we ate, talked, and cried while my friends' kids played between the pews. When it was over, we cleaned up and sent people home with the leftover food, grocery store fruit trays, bright orange deli cheddar cheese slices, and soft white grocery store bakery buns balanced in their arms as they left the church. It was both a physical act of feeding people and a gesture of care, rooted in the working-class values of the small northern city where I grew up as much as it was in the queer art of potlucks.

WHY DEATH IS AN INDUSTRY, AND WHAT WARS AND WHITENESS HAVE TO DO WITH IT

The LGBTQ+ community has a complex and intimate relationship with death. It's a proximity rooted in the violent impacts of systemic oppression: LGBTQ+ people are at higher risk of suicidal ideation and death by suicide,[273] something that has a disproportionate effect on the trans community.[274] We're the targets of violent hate crimes, which also disproportionately impact trans and gender-diverse people—especially trans women of colour and sex workers.[275] We live with the past and present legacies of the AIDS crisis, which include massive loss of life and experiences of chronic bereavement among those who survived.

In death, we and our loved ones may experience homophobia[276] and/or transphobia[277] from family members or funeral homes—a profit-motivated industry worth billions.[278] In the 1980s some funeral directors charged hundreds of dollars in unnecessary fees to care for the bodies of people who died of AIDS.[279] Even today, queer and trans people might be denied the ability to care for and honour our dying and dead in ways that align with our and our loved ones' values, identities, and cultural practices, including being unable to afford the thousands of dollars needed to hold a funeral and pay for burial or cremation, costs that are prohibitively expensive for the many

LGBTQ+ people living in poverty. These are all forms of systemic violence—a closing off of possibilities for ritual, remembrance, and healing.

The modern funeral industry is ecologically destructive, too. Typical burial or cremation practices poison the air and water with toxic chemicals and take a heavy toll on the land.[280] Each year, approximately 3.1 million litres of formaldehyde are buried along with the bodies of people laid to rest in American cemeteries, as well as 73,000 kilometres of hardwood boards, 58,500 tons of steel, and 1.5 million tons of concrete.[281] Cremation isn't much better because it consumes a lot of energy (all that heat has to come from somewhere) and emits air pollution. Indigenous, Black, and other racialized communities tend to bear a much greater burden of the health impacts of toxic contamination and pollution as a result of environmental racism. In an article on the environmental racism Black people face after death, Leanna First-Arai draws attention to the fact that many cemeteries used by the Black community are located near toxic industries or in areas prone to flooding.[282] For example, First-Arai notes that within a five-mile radius of George Floyd's grave in Pearland, Texas, there are twelve facilities releasing so many chemicals dangerous to human health they're subject to mandatory reporting by the US Environmental Protection Agency.

The history of deathcare in North America is entangled with white supremacy, misogyny, war, and capitalism. The origins of the modern funeral industry date back to the 1860s, during the US Civil War era, when approximately 620,000 soldiers died.[283] They needed a way to preserve soldiers' bodies for the long trip from the battlefield to their final resting place—that's when embalming became common, a practice popularized after Abraham Lincoln's embalmed body travelled on a funeral train through 180 cities and seven states.[284] Before then, families commonly cared for their own dead at home, work largely done by women. As historian of death and dying

Kami Fletcher explains, "When someone was dying it was the women who cared for them. When there was a confirmed death in the community, it was the women who were first called to conduct the mourning, handle the body, and organize obsequies [funeral rites]."[285]

The popularization of embalming helped turn deathcare from a community-led tradition into a profitable business. It soon became a male-dominated profession centred on trades like undertaking and casket-making. Caring for the dead was no longer something families and loved ones did at home; it was a service they purchased from a newly created industry led by men. In this way, the masculinization and professionalization of deathcare parallels the medicalization of pregnancy and birth, a process driven by white male physicians who depicted midwives as barbaric, dirty, and an evil to be controlled.[286]

It's in this history that we can find the origins of modern beliefs like the idea that dead bodies are inherently dangerous or dirty, embalming is always necessary before burial, and only funeral professionals are qualified to tend to and transport the bodies of our loved ones with the help of their specialized facilities and vehicles.

In recounting this history, it's important to point to the fact that I'm referring to beliefs and practices common among white people in North America, beliefs and practices that I now understand were foundational in shaping my understanding of what to do when someone dies. Different cultures, faith traditions, and communities have their own beliefs and practices around dying, death, and grief, and in North America those beliefs and practices exist alongside colonialism, white supremacy, and systemic oppression.

Writing on behalf of The Collective for Radical Death Studies, Kami Fletcher calls attention to how European settler colonialism has affected "the death, dying, burial [and] last rites rituals of persons of colour."[287] For example, she writes of how enslaved African and Black people were literally worked to death by white slaveholders and then denied the ability to practise their traditional deathways.[288] The

Coalition for Radical Death Studies calls on us to connect this history to the present-day realities of how systemic oppression undergirds the ways people of colour die, whether at the hands of the police or an unjust medical system, or through the cumulative health impacts of oppression.[289]

Decolonizing death requires us to centre the historical and contemporary deathways of Indigenous, Black, Latinx, Asian, and other communities of colour. For example, Black funeral traditions like homegoings, a Christian service celebrating the dead person's return to heaven, "can offer Black Americans the respect in death they don't always receive in life" and "provide refuge for the living" through careful adornment of the dead, beautiful flower arrangements, and a sense of pride and pageantry.[290] The 2013 documentary film *Homegoings* tells the story of Isaiah Owens, a Black funeral director and owner of the Owens Funeral Home, where their slogan is, "Where beauty softens your grief."[291] In addition to serving their communities, Black funeral homes played a role in the civil rights movement—in 1963, funeral director A.G. Gaston paid the $5,000 bail for Martin Luther King Jr. and Ralph Abernathy, and civil rights leaders sometimes used hearses to travel undetected.[292] If we are to queer death, we must also decolonize it by accounting for and honouring these histories and present-day practices among Indigenous, Black, Latinx, Asian, and other communities of colour.

BURY ME FURIOUSLY: QUEERNESS AND MOURNING AS COMMUNITY HEALING AND ACTIVISM

Some of my first queer teachers about death were leatherdykes I met when I was in my late twenties. They were a tight-knit group of dykes and variously gendered queers older than me who'd already had close family members and loved ones die. They'd been activists during the AIDS crisis, protesting in 1987 with the local chapter of AIDS Coalition To Unleash Power (ACT UP) when the government of British Columbia threatened to quarantine people living with AIDS. They were intimate with death in a way I wasn't then.

I saw them sit together night after night in 2009 when Catherine, a queer femme and proud leatherdyke beloved by many in the community, died unexpectedly in a plane crash. The day of Catherine's memorial, dozens of us used our bodies to block traffic so her closest mourners could carry her coffin down the street and into the community hall where her wake was held. An opera singer and a femme honour guard led the funeral procession into the same hall where Catherine had previously attended raucous play parties.

As I reflect on what it might look like to queer death, I also look to our LGBTQ+ lineages and community practices of remembrance and mourning. During the height of the AIDS crisis, the partners of people who were dying held vigils and created their own rituals when their beloveds died.[293] They washed, dressed, and visited with their bodies, held ceremonies, built altars, and organized their own memorials ranging from religious services to dances and parties.

There is an iconic photo of artist, writer, and activist David Wojnarowicz at a 1988 ACT UP action at the US Food and Drug Administration (FDA). He's wearing a black leather jacket with a pink triangle on the back; painted overtop in bold white lettering are the words, "If I die of AIDS, forget burial—just drop my body on the steps of the FDA." A year later, in the essay "Postcards from America: X Rays from Hell," he wrote:

> I imagine what it would be like if friends had a demonstration each time a lover or a friend or a stranger died of AIDS. I imagine what it would be like if, each time a lover, friend or stranger died of this disease, their friends, lovers or neighbours would take the dead body

and drive with it in a car a hundred miles an hour to washington d.c. and blast through the gates of the white house and come to screeching halt before the entrance and dump their lifeless form on the front steps. It would be comforting to see those friends, neighbours, lovers and strangers mark time and place and history in such a public way.[294]

In October 1992, ACT UP organized a funeral procession through the streets of Washington, DC, to protest twelve years of the US government's genocidal AIDS policy.[295] It began at a nearby display of the AIDS Memorial Quilt, the group of marchers swelling in size from hundreds to thousands of people by the time they reached the White House.

There's archival footage of this procession, called the *Ashes Action*, online.[296] People march with silver urns and small cardboard boxes full of ashes held aloft in their hands, a solemn drumbeat sounding out in the background as they take over the streets. At the end of the march, they pour the ashes of the loved ones they had lost to AIDS on the White House lawn through the tall black iron fence encircling the building. Cops on horseback hover nearby as the protestors chant, "Shame! Shame! Shame!" over and over. During this action, Wojnarowicz's partner Tom Rauffenbart scattered some of his lover's ashes on the White House lawn.[297] David Robinson, whose partner Warren Krause's death inspired the action, describes in an interview being motivated to show the truth of what was happening: "*Don't pretty this up in any way*. What has come out of this epidemic? It's ashes, it's bone chips."[298]

A month later, in November 1992, ACT UP held a political funeral for Mark Lowe Fisher. They carried his body in an open casket shielded by black umbrellas through the rainy streets of New York, New York, to the Bush campaign headquarters on the eve of election day. "Bury me furiously," Fisher wrote before his death, "I want my own funeral to be fierce and defiant, to make the public statement that my death from AIDS is a form of political assassination."[299] At the funeral, a banner from a previous ACT UP action Fisher had participated in—a die-in near George H.W. Bush's vacation home in Kennebunkport, Maine—was strewn across Fisher's coffin. The banner "listed the specific steps that George Bush could take, as president, to fight AIDS," demands that went unheeded.[300]

In July 1993, ACT UP organized a political funeral for Tim Bailey, bringing his body to Washington, DC, in an effort to honour Bailey's wish that he be placed in front of the White House. There, they were met by FBI agents, undercover police, park police, and riot police who violently sought to prevent the protest. They ended up in a five-hour standoff with law enforcement, ACT UP members blockading the van with Bailey's body in it and fighting back when the police tried taking Bailey's casket out of the vehicle. As ACT UP member Ron Goldberg explained, this action "was very much about, literally, bringing the bodies of our dead to where we thought the blame [lay] and making that quantifiable ... *Here's a dead body—this was someone who we loved, who we valued.*"[301]

I also think of the more recent example of Andrew Henderson (a.k.a. Glamdrew), a twenty-eight-year-old queer artist in Winnipeg who was diagnosed with incurable cancer and, in 2016, decided to cocreate *Taking It to the Grave*, a performance that was both a living funeral and community ritual.[302] Together with collaborators Eroca Nicols, Carly Boyce, and Mars Gradiva, Glamdrew invited participants to dance on a glitter-bedecked dance floor, give themselves manicures at a nail art station, and—perhaps most powerfully—confess the secrets, regrets, or baggage they wanted him to take to the grave.

Together, Glamdrew and each confessor would create an image that represented what the person wanted to let go of. Boyce would then tattoo that image on Glamdrew's body so he could *literally* take it to the grave. I wasn't able to attend this performance—I live thousands of kilometres away—but I still think about it years later because it offered me a vision into something I didn't yet know was possible: a way to turn dying into art and create space for personal and community healing.

DEATHCARE AS IMAGINATION AND RECLAMATION

Death is inevitable, and being confronted with its reality can feel sad, scary, or overwhelming. When I think back to when my mom died, I still feel grief and regret that I wasn't able to turn that final moment at her bedside into a more intentional ritual of connection and care for her. It felt impossible for me at the time, all alone in that hospital room with no one to help or guide me.

But there can be beauty and healing in death, too. Queerness and queer community helped me find my way through death back then. They offered me a path through my grief and into healing. Now, as I contemplate my own inevitable end, I find comfort and inspiration in knowing that I can queer my own death, too. The queering of my death could be a final gift I offer to the beloved community I leave behind.

The notion of queering my own death feels like an act of radical imagination and a reclamation of practices my ancestors would've carried out.

Fortunately, I'm not alone in thinking about transforming death: there's a whole death-positive movement made up of people both within and outside of the death and funeral industries who are working toward change and trying to open up the conversation about dying and death. The tenets of this movement include breaking the culture of silence around death through open conversations and advance planning, empowering people to care for their own dead if they want to, and minimizing the environmental harms of death.[303]

The death-positive movement centres on confronting fear, shame, denial, silence, and repressive cultural norms in the service of honouring people's wishes and identities through all phases of their lives—including when we die. That seems like a pretty queer sentiment to me!

Queering death also feels like a way to push back at a capitalistic, environmentally destructive funeral industry. As someone committed to health and healing and whose work is deeply informed by disability justice, I don't want my death or the deaths of my loved ones to make other people or the land sick. Thankfully, there's a growing number of people and groups working to expand our options through practices like green funerals and, thanks to Recompose, a queer-led company in Seattle, people composting (it's more beautiful and sacred than it sounds, I promise).

I didn't know until recently that it was possible to care for our own dead at home or that it's legal to hold a home funeral in both Canada and the United States. There's a whole movement of home funeral practitioners and advocates—led largely by older women—who are teaching and supporting people to care for their own dead. Funeral director Lucinda Herring vividly portrays her experiences with this work in her book *Reimagining Death*. I was moved by the stories she shared, including those of her own mother's and father's deaths and home funerals at their beloved homestead in Alabama, where their families, communities, and the natural world came together to mark their passings.[304]

When I read the stories in *Reimagining Death*, something healed in me. For years I'd carried a heartbreak about not being able to wash, dress, and care for my mom's body when she died. I felt scared and overwhelmed by the prospect and I didn't have anyone to help me with this final act of care. Reading stories from other people who'd been supported to care for their loved ones in this way was a balm. It felt comforting and empowering to learn that I have different choices and a whole community of people to look to for guidance through organizations like the Canadian Integrative Network for Death Education and Alternatives and the National Home Funeral Alliance in the United States.

This kind of thing isn't for everyone—for example, in an interview Kami Fletcher points out the importance of embalming in many Black funeral traditions—yet she also emphasizes the liberatory potential of home funerals for groups like the queer and trans community as a way to sidestep the commercial funeral industry and discrimination from our dead loved ones' families of origin.[305]

PUT ME IN THE LIVING ROOM AND COVER ME WITH FLOWERS

I want us to become more comfortable and intimate with death, not because we constantly fear that our lives are in peril or because too many of our beloveds have died, but because we trust that it can offer healing amid the pain of loss. I want queer and trans folks to have the information and skills we need to be able to talk openly about our own wishes: What would a good death look and feel like for you? What do you want to happen to your body after you die? How do you want us to mourn and celebrate you? I want us to have what writer Aisha Adkins calls a "death buddy," a trusted friend with whom you can talk openly about your wishes, fears, and questions about death.[306]

Perhaps we can take inspiration from ninety-year-old queer activist and former nurse Shatzi Weisberger, who hosted her own death party.[307] There, a hundred guests joined her in decorating her biodegradable cardboard coffin with glitter while they ate prawn cocktails, drank wine, got temporary tattoos, and listened to a performance by the Brooklyn Women's Chorus. She held this party as a way to get people talking about death, often a taboo topic in a death-phobic culture.

I want there to be queer and trans community–led death collectives where people have the resources, support, and information they need to care for their dying and their beloved dead—or plan for their own deaths—in ways that feel meaningful, affirming, and culturally safe to them. I want Indigenous, Black, Latinx, Asian, and other communities of colour to have access to deathcare that reflects and centres their cultural and spiritual traditions and practices, and affirms their queer and trans identities. I want everybody who wants one to have access to a queer- and/or trans-affirming death doula.

I want there to be community deathcare funds that help cover all the costs associated with someone's death. I never want to see another queer or trans person have to do a GoFundMe for a funeral again. I want all queer and trans folks who need to access palliative or hospice care to be cared for by providers who practise from a place deeply rooted in disability justice, antiracism, and a fierce commitment to honouring and celebrating queer and trans lives.

I want people to have the choice of medically assisted death because it's a way to enact their desires and assert their bodily sovereignty, not because it feels like a grim and unavoidable alternative to living in an ableist society where they aren't able to receive all the care, resources, and support they need to flourish in life.

I want all queer and trans people to live long, joyful lives surrounded by beloved community and when our times come, I want us to die well and to be loved, cared for, and honoured in death as we were in life.

One of the biggest gifts my experience of queering death has given me is the opportunity to dream differently about what my own might look like:

When I die, I want my beloveds to wash and anoint my body with oils. Dress me in something beautiful. Put me on dry ice and place me in a comfortable spot where people can visit with me. Adorn that space with flowers and photos. Make it feel sacred. Pray over me. Sing, laugh, cry. Remember to breathe, eat, and drink water. Now that my chest no longer rises and falls, practise being in the new quality of silence that accompanies the cessation of my breath and voice. Whisper loving words to me. Pass me a note.

Gather together so you aren't alone in your grief. Share a meal with each other. Tell stories. Howl at the moon. Choose solitude when you need it (I'll be there with you). Have a ritual. Cast spells to guide me across the threshold between this life and whatever is on the other side. Spend time with me until you're ready to let me go. When that time comes, wrap my body in a linen shroud, cover me in flowers, and give me back to the earth.

I am here, on this threshold, ready to become your fierce femme ancestor. Remember me and remember that my love for you is eternal and spans generations. Keep a picture of me on your altar. Light a candle. Leave an offering. Say my name when you need me. Know that I will keep loving and fighting for you, long after I draw my last breath.

ACKNOWLEDGMENTS

Writing is an embodied, relational, and place-based act. Every word of this book was written on stolen Indigenous lands. Today, I live as a white settler and uninvited visitor on the traditional, ancestral, shared territories of the xʷməθkʷəy̓əm (Musqueam), Sḵwx̱wú7mesh (Squamish), and səlilwətaʔɬ (Tsleil-Waututh) First Nations. As a person of Scottish and Irish ancestry, I am in a continuous process of learning and practising what it means to be a respectful guest on lands that don't belong to me. This commitment is threaded through my everyday actions, in my work as a writer, activist, and advocate, and in how I parent a white child who, like me, was born on stolen Indigenous lands.

Every aspect of creating *The Care We Dream Of* was guided by a core intention: *Let this book, and the process of creating it, be a spell of healing and transformation, rooted in love*. I wanted to create this book in a way that was reflective of the liberatory visions of health and healing that animate it. This commitment became even more important when the COVID-19 pandemic was declared early in the process of creating it. It is a book rooted in queer care and relationships, and I offer my deep gratitude and fierce femme love to all the people who share their words and ideas in these pages: Alexander McClelland and Zoë Dodd, Anita "Durt" O'Shea, Blyth Barnow, Carly Boyce, Dawn Serra, Hannah Kia, jaye simpson, Jillian Christmas, Joshua Wales, Kai Cheng Thom, Leah Lakshmi Piepzna-Samarasinha, Ronica Mukerjee, Sand C. Chang, and Sean Saifa Wall.

I offer my thanks and abiding love and loyalty to the team at Arsenal Pulp Press. This is my third book with Arsenal over a ten-year period, and I keep returning to them for a reason: because I trust deeply in their commitment to publishing beautiful, radical queer and trans books with integrity and care. Brian, Robert, Cynara,

Jaiden, Jaz, and Catharine: thank you for everything you do, and for the spirit with which you do it. Thank you to Shirarose Wilensky for her skilful and caring editorial guidance and for believing in this project from the beginning. I'm also grateful to Erin Parker for her insightful, compassionate, and responsive editorial support.

Leah Lakshmi Piepzna-Samarasinha was my writing coach throughout the process of creating *The Care We Dream Of*. We spent hours workshopping my writing, talking through ideas, laughing, crying, and generally loving on each other for the two years it took to bring this book into being. Leah, there aren't enough Coach Taylor memes in the world to show you how grateful I am for the experience of working with you. It made me a better, more honest writer, helped me find pleasure and ease in the work, and taught me so much about what it looks and feels like to put disability justice into practice.

I'm grateful to artist Tiaré Lani Kela Jung for creating the beautiful art that graces the cover and interior of this book. Thank you for engaging so fully with the purpose and ideas at the core of *The Care We Dream Of* and for translating them into such gorgeous and meaningful images.

In an essay on the importance of finding trusted early readers, author Sheila Heti wrote, "Art is made in the space between the artist and their early, chosen readers, a space that is filled with love, and with the pleasure of mutually solving a puzzle with care." Thank you to all the early readers who gave me the gift of your feedback on all or parts of this manuscript while it was still taking shape: Amber Dawn, Carolyn Camman, Claire Bodkin, Gisele da Silva, Hannah McGregor, Hazel Jane Plante, Harper Keenan, Kendra Marks, Meenakshi Mannoe, Michael V. Smith, Ryan Backer, Tharuna Abbu, and Timothy Keyes. Thanks to Alexander McClelland, Eli Manning, Rod Knight, and Travis Salway for answering my questions and generously sharing your research expertise. Thanks also to Alexis Pauline Gumbs and Hil Malatino, whose work I admire so deeply, for the gift of being able to use your words as the epigraph to *The Care We Dream Of*.

Finally, thank you to my family: Scout, Linden, Jen, and Rowan. You offer me the care I dream of every day in how we create home and family together. I couldn't have written this book without your love and support.

ENDNOTES

INTRODUCTION

1   Bobbie Harro, "The Cycle of Liberation" in *Readings for Diversity and Social Justice*, ed. M. Adams et al. (New York: Routledge, 2000), quoted in Maya Schenwar and Victoria Law, *Prison by Any Other Name: The Harmful Consequences of Popular Reform* (New York: The New Press, 2021), 23.

2   Health care workers and scholars have engaged with the idea of liberation in health and health care—for example, liberation medicine as conceptualized and practised by Doctors for Global Health (Lanny Smith with Ken Hilsbos, "Liberation Medicine: Health & Justice," Doctors for Global Health, accessed May 20, 2021, https://www.dghonline.org/content/liberation-medicine-health-justice) and the idea of health as liberation that bioethicist Alastair V. Campbell explores in his book of the same name (Alastair V. Campbell, *Health as Liberation: Medicine, Theology, and the Quest for Justice* [Cleveland: The Pilgrim Press, 1995]), both of which are informed by liberation theology. More recently, the organizers and participants of the 2019 Liberation Health Convergence engaged with the concept of liberation with a focus on developing a community/network of liberationist health care workers (Nikisha Khare and Nanky Rai, "Health Care toward Liberation," *Briarpatch*, November 25, 2020, https://briarpatchmagazine.com/articles/view/health-care-toward-liberation).

3   Dean Spade, *Normal Life: Administrative Violence, Critical Trans Politics, and the Limits of Law* (Brooklyn: South End Press, 2011), 20.

4   European Union Agency for Fundamental Rights, *EU LGBT Survey: Main Results* (Vienna: European Union, 2014); Sandy E. James, Jody L. Herman, Susan Rankin, Mara Keisling, Lisa Mottet, and Ma'ayan Anafi, *The Report of the 2015 U.S. Transgender Survey* (Washington: National Center for Transgender Equality, 2016); Lambda Legal, *When Health Care Isn't Caring* (New York: Lambda Legal, 2010); Shabab Ahmed Mirza and Caitlin Rooney, "Discrimination Prevents LGBTQ People from Accessing Health Care," Center for American Progress, January 18, 2018, https://www.americanprogress.org/issues/lgbtq-rights/news/2018/01/18/445130/discrimination-prevents-lgbtq-people-accessing-health-care/.

5   Human Rights Campaign, "Health Disparities among Bisexual People," accessed May 21, 2021, https://www.hrc.org/resources/health-disparities-among-bisexual-people.

6   Kat Butler, Adryen Yak, and Albina Veltman, "'Progress in Medicine Is Slower to Happen': Qualitative Insights into How Trans and Gender Nonconform-

ing Medical Students Navigate Cisnormative Medical Cultures at Canadian Training Programs," *Academic Medicine* 94, no. 11 (2019): 1757–65; Michele J. Eliason, Suzanne L. Dibble, and Patricia A. Robertson, "Lesbian, Gay, Bisexual, and Transgender (LGBT) Physicians' Experiences in the Workplace," *Journal of Homosexuality* 58, no. 10 (2011): 1355–71; Julia M. Przedworski et al., "A Comparison of the Mental Health and Well-Being of Sexual Minority and Heterosexual First-Year Medical Students: A Report from the Medical Student CHANGE Study," *Academic Medicine* 90, no. 5 (2015): 652–59; Elizabeth A. Samuels, Dowin H. Boatright, Ambrose H. Wong, Laura D. Cramer, Mayur M. Desai, Michael T. Solotke, Darin Latimore, and Cary P. Gross, "Association between Sexual Orientation, Mistreatment, and Burnout among US Medical Students," *JAMA Network Open* 4, no. 2 (2021): e2036136, doi:10.1001/jama networkopen.2020.36136.

7   Greta R. Bauer, Ayden I. Scheim, Madeline B. Deutsch, and Carys Massarella, "Reported Emergency Department Avoidance, Use, and Experiences of Transgender Persons in Ontario, Canada: Results from a Respondent-Driven Sampling Survey," *Annals of Emergency Medicine* 63, no. 6 (2014): 713–20; Greta R. Bauer, Xuchen Zong, Ayden I. Scheim, Rebecca Hammond, and Amardeep Thind, "Factors Impacting Transgender Patients' Discomfort with Their Family Physicians: A Respondent-Driven Sampling Survey," *PLoS ONE* 10, no. 12: e0145046, doi:10.1371/journal.pone.0145046; Beth A. Clark, Jaimie F. Veale, Devon Greyson, and Elizabeth Saewyc, "Primary Care Access and Foregone Care: A Survey of Transgender Adolescents and Young Adults," *Family Practice* 35, no. 3 (2018): 302–6.

8   andrea bennett, *Like a Boy but Not a Boy: Navigating Life, Mental Health, and Parenthood outside the Gender Binary* (Vancouver: Arsenal Pulp Press, 2020), 52–53.

9   Myrl Beam, *Gay, Inc.: The Nonprofitization of Queer Politics* (Minneapolis: University of Minnesota Press, 2018), 164.

10 Museum of the City of New York, "When Existence Is Resistance: Transgender Activism, 1969–2019," Activist New York lesson plan, accessed May 20, 2021, https://activistnewyork.mcny.org/sites/default/files/LessonPlanTrans Activism_0.pdf.

11 Rebecca Belmore, "Twelve Angry Crinolines," accessed April 19, 2021, https://www.rebeccabelmore.com/twelve-angry-crinolines/.

12 Wanda Nanibush, "An Interview with Rebecca Belmore," *Decolonization: Indigeneity, Education & Society* 3, no. 1 (2014): 213–17.

13 Reuters, "Three More of Queen's Cousins Kept in Asylum," *Los Angeles Times*, April 7, 1987, accessed April 19, 2021, https://www.latimes.com/archives/la-xpm -1987-04-07-mn-323-story.html.

14 Christopher Hume, "Women Artists Claim Plight Parallels Royal Incarcerations," *Toronto Star*, July 17, 1987.

15 Theresa Stewart-Ambo and K. Wayne Yang, "Beyond Land Acknowledgment in Settler Institutions," *Social Text* 39, no. 1 (2021): 21–46.

16 Eve Tuck and K. Wayne Yang, "Decolonization Is Not a Metaphor," *Decolonization: Indigeneity, Education & Society* 1, no. 1 (2012): 1–40.

QUEER ALCHEMY

17 Lex Non Scripta, "A Few Years Ago I Was Working On a Series Of," *Tumblr* (blog), December 19, 2012, https://lexnonscripta.tumblr.com/post/38346657137/a-few-years-ago-i-was-working-on-a-series-of.

18 Queer Nation NY, "Queer Nation NY History," 2016, https://queernationny.org/history.

19 Associated Press, "100 Arrested at ACT UP Protest of CDC's AIDS Definition," December 4, 1990, https://apnews.com/article/a7dbdbb360dc0ff1586fbfaa02400413.

20 ACT UP New York, "Actions," accessed November 11, 2020, https://actupny.com/actions/; Andrea Anderson, "Demonstrating Discontent: May 21, 1990," *The Scientist*, July 16, 2017, https://www.the-scientist.com/foundations/demonstrating-discontent-may-21-1990-31227.

21 amfAR, "HIV/AIDS: Snapshots of an Epidemic," accessed November 11, 2020, https://www.amfar.org/thirty-years-of-HIV/AIDS-snapshots-of-an-epidemic/.

22 Alisa Bierria, "Pursuing a Radical Anti-violence Agenda inside/outside a Non-profit Structure," in *The Revolution Will Not Be Funded: Beyond the Non-profit Industrial Complex*, ed. INCITE! Women of Color Against Violence (Durham: Duke University Press, 2017), 158.

23 Aurora Levins Morales, "Building Radical Soil," in *Medicine Stories: Essays for Radicals* (Durham: Duke University Press, 2019), 209.

24 Zena Sharman, interview with Hannah McGregor (host), "A Trojan Horse of Radical Values with Zena Sharman," *Secret Feminist Agenda* (podcast), March 1, 2019, https://secretfeministagenda.com/2019/03/01/episode-3-20-a-trojan-horse-of-radical-values-with-zena-sharman/.

25 *Merriam-Webster*, "Alchemy," accessed October 27, 2020, https://www.merriam-webster.com/dictionary/alchemy.

26 adrienne maree brown, "Dream beyond the Wounds," *Ding Magazine*, accessed April 26, 2021, https://dingdingding.org/issue-2/dream-beyond-the-wounds/.

27 Hil Malatino, "Tough Breaks: Trans Rage and the Cultivation of Resilience," *Hypatia* 34, no. 1 (2019): 133.

28 Rob Cover, "Resilience," in *Critical Concepts in Queer Studies and Education*, eds. Nelson M. Rodriguez, Wayne J. Martino, Jennifer C. Ingrey, and Edward Brockenbrough (New York: Palgrave Macmillan, 2016), 351–60.

29 Sins Invalid, *Skin, Tooth, and Bone: The Basis of Movement Is Our People*, 2nd ed., 2019, 12.

30 Leah Lakshmi Piepzna-Samarasinha, *Care Work: Dreaming Disability Justice* (Vancouver: Arsenal Pulp Press, 2018), 22.

31 Liat Ben-Moshe, *Decarcerating Disability: Deinstitutionalization and Prison Abolition* (Minneapolis: University of Minnesota Press, 2020), 125.

32 Audre Lorde, "Learning from the 60s," *Black Past*, August 12, 2012, https://www.blackpast.org/african-american-history/1982-audre-lorde-learning-60s/.

33 Masti Khor and Chanelle Gallant, *Kink and Trauma: BDSM as Self-Care for Survivors*, self-published zine (n.d.), 17.

34 Sins Invalid, *Skin, Tooth, and Bone*, 19.

CRIPPING HEALING

35 Aurora Levins Morales, Qwo-Li Driskill, and Leah Lakshmi Piepzna-Samarasinha, "Sweet Dark Places: Letters to Gloria Anzaldúa on Disability, Creativity, and the Coatlicue State," in *El Mundo Zurdo 2: Selected Works from the 2010 Meeting of the Society for the Study of Gloria Anzaldúa*, eds. Norma Alarcón, Rita E. Urquijo-Ruiz, and Sonia Saldívar-Hull (San Francisco: Aunt Lute Books, 2012), 84.

36 Sins Invalid, *Skin, Tooth, and Bone: The Basis of Movement Is Our People*, 2nd ed., 2019, 12.

37 Disability Rights Education & Defense Fund, "Stacey Park Milbern: May 19, 1987–May 19, 2020," accessed June 16, 2021, https://dredf.org/2020/05/20/stacey-milbern-park/.

38 Audre Lorde, "Learning from the 60s," in *Sister Outsider: Essays and Speeches* (Ithaca: Crossing Press, 1982), 137.

39 "Crip Lineages, Crip Futures: A Conversation with Stacey Milbern," in Leah Lakshmi Piepzna-Samarasinha, *Care Work: Dreaming Disability Justice* (Vancouver: Arsenal Pulp, 2018), 240.

40 Alex Haagaard, "Notes on Temporal Inaccessibility," March 12, 2021, https://alexhaagaard.medium.com/notes-on-temporal-inaccessibility-28ebcdf1b6d6.

41 Eli Clare, *Brilliant Imperfection: Grappling with Cure* (Durham: Duke University Press, 2017), 25. Quotations from this book reprinted with permission.

42 Ibid., 85.

43 Ibid., 90.

44 Ibid., 13.

45 Ibid., 61.

46 Joseph Shapiro, "One Man's COVID-19 Death Raises the Worst Fears of Many People with Disabilities," NPR, July 31, 2020, https://www.npr.org/2020/07/31/896882268/one-mans-COVID-19-death-raises-the-worst-fears-of-many-people-with-disabilities.

47 International Community Health Services, "I Feel Like I'm with Family," accessed April 30, 2021, https://www.ichs.com/i-feel-like-im-with-family/.

THE SYSTEM ISN'T BROKEN, IT'S WORKING AS DESIGNED

48 World Health Organization, *Everybody's Business: Strengthening Health Systems to Improve Health Outcomes: WHO's Framework for Action* (Geneva: World Health Organization, 2007), 2.

49 Canadian Medical Association, "Proportion of Physicians Who Receive 90+% of Their Income from Specific Methods of Remuneration," accessed March 14, 2021, https://www.cma.ca/sites/default/files/pdf/Physician%20Data/38-Remuneration-e.pdf.

50 Danielle Martin, *Better Now: Six Big Ideas to Improve Health Care for All Canadians* (Toronto: Penguin Canada, 2017).

51 Lorne Brown and Doug Taylor, "The Birth of Medicare: From Saskatchewan's Breakthrough to Canada-Wide Coverage," *Canadian Dimension*, July 3, 2012, https://canadiandimension.com/articles/view/the-birth-of-medicare.

52 Ibid.

53 Danielle Martin, Ashley P. Miller, Amélie Quesnel-Vallée, Nadine R. Caron, Bilkis Vissandjée, and Gregory P. Marchildon, "Canada's Universal Health-Care System: Achieving Its Potential," *Lancet* 391, no. 10131 (2018): 1718–35.

54 Ibid.

55 Graham Hudson, Rebecca Cheff, Mylini Saposan, and Arnav Agarwal, "COVID-19 Exposing Cracks in Our Universal Healthcare," *Healthy Debate*, October 22, 2020, https://healthydebate.ca/opinions/COVID-19-cracks-in-healthcare/.

56 Sandy E. James, Jody L. Herman, Susan Rankin, Mara Keisling, Lisa Mottet, and Ma'ayan Anafi, *The Report of the 2015 U.S. Transgender Survey* (Washington: National Center for Transgender Equality, 2016).

57 Eli Clare, *Brilliant Imperfection: Grappling with Cure* (Durham: Duke University Press, 2017), 28.

58 Emily Allen Paine, "'Fat Broken Arm Syndrome': Negotiating Risk, Stigma, and Weight Bias in LGBTQ Healthcare," *Social Science & Medicine* 270 (2021): 113609.

59 Heidi L. Janz, "Ableism: The Undiagnosed Malady Afflicting Medicine," *Canadian Medical Association Journal*, 191, no. 17 (2019): E478–E479, doi:10.1503/cmaj.180903.

60 Marc Gaspar, Travis Salway, and Daniel Grace, "Ambivalence and the Biopolitics of HIV Pre-exposure Prophylaxis (PrEP) Implementation," *Social Theory & Health* (2021): doi:10.1057/s41285-020-00154-w.

61 Merlin Chowkwanyun, "The New Left and Public Health: The Health Policy Advisory Center, Community Organizing, and the Big Business of Health, 1967–1975," *American Journal of Public Health* 101, no. 2 (2011): 238–49; People's Health Movement, "Healthcare in the USA: Understanding the Medical-Industrial Complex," *Global Health Watch 5* (2018), accessed March 24, 2021, https://phmovement.org/wp-content/uploads/2018/07/B3.pdf; Barbara and John Ehrenreich, *The American Health Empire: Power, Profits and Politics* (New York: Random House, 1970).

62 Anjali Taneja, Cara Page, and Susan Raffo, "Healing Histories: Disrupting the Medical Industrial Complex," September 13, 2019, https://www.susanraffo.com/blog/healing-histories-disrupting-the-medical-industrial-complex-1.

63 Mia Mingus, "Medical Industrial Complex Visual," *Leaving Evidence* (blog), February 6, 2015, https://leavingevidence.wordpress.com/2015/02/06/medical-industrial-complex-visual/.

64 Ibid.

65 Mordecai Cohen Ettinger, "Understanding and Transforming the Medical-Industrial Complex, Part 2: Session 5," Health Justice Commons course lecture (via Zoom), March 25, 2020.

66 Anjali Taneja and Cara Page, "Healing Histories: Disrupting the Medical Industrial Complex, and Casa de Salud," Keynote address, Doctors for Global Health 25th Annual General Assembly, August 9, 2020, https://www.youtube.com/watch?v=Jq_btWV-mZc.

67 Marsha Barber, "How the Medical School Admissions Process Is Skewed," *University Affairs*, November 30, 2016, https://www.universityaffairs.ca/features/feature-article/medical-school-admissions-process-skewed/; Kwang Jin Choi, Hyo Jung Tak, Clark Bach, Cathleen Trias, Huma Warsi, Joseph Abraham, and John D. Yoon, "Characteristics of Medical Students with Physician Relatives: A National Study," *MedEdPublish*, 7, [1], 30 (2018): doi:10.15694/mep.2018.0000030.1; Marc J. Kahn and Ernest J. Sneed, "Promoting the Affordability of Medical Education to Groups Underrepresented in the Profession: The Other Side of the Equation," *AMA Journal of Ethics*, 17, no. 2 (2015): 172–75.

68   Jay Youngclaus and Lindsay Roskovensky, "An Updated Look at the Economic Diversity of U.S. Medical Students," AAMC *Analysis in Brief* 18, no. 5 (2018): https://www.aamc.org/media/9596/download.

69   Association of American Medical Colleges, "Matriculating Student Questionnaire: 2020 All Schools Summary Report," accessed May 28, 2021, https://www.aamc.org/media/50081/download; Tricia Pendergrast (@traependergrast), Twitter thread, July 22, 2020, 7:27 a.m., https://twitter.com/traependergrast/status/1285945961173458945.

70   Rishad Khan, Tavis Apramian, Joel Hosung Kang, Jeffrey Gustafson, and Shannon Sibbald, "Demographic and Socioeconomic Characteristics of Canadian Medical Students: A Cross-Sectional Study," BMC *Medical Education* 20, no. 151 (2020): doi:10.1186/s12909-020-02056-x; Tyler Pitre, Alexander Thomas, Kyle Evans, Aaron Jones, Margo Mountjoy, and Andrew P. Costa, "The Influence of Income on Medical School Admissions in Canada: A Retrospective Cohort Study," BMC *Medical Education* 20, no. 209 (2020): doi:10.1186/s12909-020-02126-0.

71   Max Jordan Nguemeni Tiako, Eugenia C. South, and Victor Ray, "Medical Schools as Racialized Organizations: A Primer," *Annals of Internal Medicine* (2021): doi:10.7326/M21-0369.

72   American Association of Medical Colleges, "Diversity in Medicine: Facts and Figures 2019," accessed May 1, 2021, https://www.aamc.org/data-reports/workforce/report/diversity-medicine-facts-and-figures-2019; Lanair Amaad Lett, H. Moses Murdock, Whitney U. Orji, Jaya Aysola, and Ronnie Sebro, "Trends in Racial/Ethnic Representation among US Medical Students," *JAMA Network Open* 2, no. 9 (2019): e1910490, doi:10.1001/jamanetworkopen.2019.10490.

73   Khan et al., "Demographic and Socioeconomic Characteristics of Canadian Medical Students."

74   Lisa M. Meeks and Kurt R. Herzer, "Prevalence of Self-Disclosed Disability among Medical Students in US Allopathic Medical Schools," *Journal of the American Medical Association* 316, no. 21 (2016): 2271–72; Omar S. Haque, Michael A. Stein, and Amelia Marvit, "Physician, Heal Thy Double Stigma—Doctors with Mental Illness and Structural Barriers to Disclosure," *New England Journal of Medicine* 384, no. 10 (2021): 888–91.

75   Nanky Rai, *Uprooting Medical Violence: Building an Integrated Anti-oppression Framework for Primary Health Care*, accessed May 1, 2021, https://docs.google.com/document/d/1fVkVw2vOSF_TowE3cmfo_wM4s6_Yp74Lzhz2sUUj4iA/edit.

76   Edward C. Halperin, Jay A. Perman, and Emery A. Wilson, "Abraham Flexner of Kentucky, His Report, Medical Education in the United States and Canada, and the Historical Questions Raised by the Report," *Academic Medicine* 85, no. 2 (2010), 205.

77 AFL-CIO, "The 1892 Homestead Strike," accessed March 28, 2021, https://aflcio .org/about/history/labor-history-events/1892-homestead-strike.

78 Columbia University Libraries Rare Book and Manuscript Library, "Philanthropy of Andrew Carnegie," accessed March 28, 2021, https://library.columbia.edu/ libraries/rbml/units/carnegie/andrew.html.

79 Andrea Smith, "Introduction," in *The Revolution Will Not Be Funded: Beyond the Non-profit Industrial Complex*, eds. INCITE! Women of Color Against Violence (Durham: Duke University Press, 2017), 4.

80 Halperin, Perman, and Wilson, "Abraham Flexner of Kentucky," 208.

81 James L. Madara, "Reckoning with Medicine's History of Racism," American Medical Association, February 17, 2021, https://www.ama-assn.org/about/leader ship/reckoning-medicine-s-history-racism.

82 National Medical Association, "History," accessed May 30, 2021, https://www. nmanet.org/page/History.

83 Michael Helquist, *Marie Equi: Radical Politics and Outlaw Passions* (Corvallis: Oregon State University Press, 2015), 85.

84 Moya Bailey, "The Flexner Report: Standardizing Medical Students through Region-, Gender-, and Race-Based Hierarchies," *American Journal of Law and Medicine* 43, no. 2–3 (2017): 213.

85 Ann Steinecke and Charles Terrell, "Progress for Whose Future? The Impact of the Flexner Report on Medical Education for Racial and Ethnic Minority Physicians in the United States," *Academic Medicine* 85, no. 2 (2010): 238.

86 Halperin, Perman, and Wilson, "Abraham Flexner of Kentucky," 206.

87 Ibid., 209.

88 Steinecke and Terrell, "Progress for Whose Future?" 238.

89 Bailey, "The Flexner Report," 214.

90 Halperin, Perman, and Wilson, "Abraham Flexner of Kentucky," 209.

91 Frank W. Stahnisch and Marja Verhoef, "The Flexner Report of 1910 and Its Impact on Complementary and Alternative Medicine and Psychiatry in North America in the 20th Century," *Evidence-Based Complementary and Alternative Medicine*, 2012, doi:10.1155/2012/647896.

92 Kendall M. Campbell, Irma Corral, Jhojana L. Infante Linares, and Dmitry Tumin, "Projected Estimates of African American Medical Graduates of Closed Historically Black Medical Schools," *JAMA Network Open* 3, no. 8 (2020): e2015220, doi:10.1001/jamanetworkopen.2020.15220.

93 Shari L. Barkin, Elena Fuentes-Afflick, Jeffrey P. Brosco, and Arleen M. Tuchman, "Unintended Consequences of the Flexner Report: Women in Pediatrics," *Pediatrics* 126, no. 6 (2010): 1055–57, doi:10.1542/peds.2010-2050.

94   American Association of Medical Colleges, "2018–2019 The State of Women in Academic Medicine: Exploring Pathways to Equity," accessed June 2, 2021, https://www.aamc.org/data-reports/data/2018-2019-state-women -academic-medicine-exploring-pathways-equity; American Association of Medical Colleges, "The Majority of U.S. Medical Students Are Women, New Data Show," December 9, 2019, https://www.aamc.org/news-insights/press -releases/majority-us-medical-students-are-women-new-data-show.

95   Susan P. Phillips, Jenna Webber, Stephan Imbeau, Tanis Quaife, Deanna Hagan, Marion Maar, and Jacques Abourbih, "Sexual Harassment of Canadian Medical Students: A National Survey," EClinical Medicine 7, no. 7 (2019): 15–20; Emily A. Vargas, Sheila T. Brassel, Lilia M. Cortina, Isis H. Settles, Timothy R.B. Johnson, and Reshma Jagsi, "#MedToo: A Large-Scale Examination of the Incidence and Impact of Sexual Harassment of Physicians and Other Faculty at an Academic Medical Center," Journal of Women's Health 29, no. 1 (2020): 13–20.

96   Kat Butler, Adryen Yak, and Albina Veltman, "'Progress in Medicine Is Slower to Happen': Qualitative Insights into How Trans and Gender Nonconforming Medical Students Navigate Cisnormative Medical Cultures at Canadian Training Programs," Academic Medicine 94, no. 11 (2019): 1757–65.

97   Bailey, "The Flexner Report," 210.

98   Canadian Public Health Association, "What Is Public Health?," accessed May 28, 2021, https://www.cpha.ca/what-public-health.

99   Jayne Malenfant, Colin Hastings, Katarina Bogosavljevic, Aziz Choudry, and Alexander McClelland, We Can't Police Our Way Out of the Pandemic: Lessons for Abolition, accessed May 1, 2021, https://documentcloud.adobe.com/link/ review?uri=urn:aaid:scds:US:f4a8f4cb-39b3-43ba-8a74-f0d760722cb1.

100 Canadian Civil Liberties Association, Stay Off the Grass: COVID-19 and Law Enforcement in Canada (Toronto: CCLA, 2020), https://ccla.org/cclanewsite/ wp-content/uploads/2020/06/2020-06-24-Stay-Off-the-Grass-COVID19-and -Law-Enforcement-in-Canada1.pdf.

101 Canadian Civil Liberties Association and the Policing the Pandemic Mapping Project, "By the Numbers: The Second Wave of COVID-19 Law Enforcement in Canada," May 12, 2021, https://ccla.org/cclanewsite/wp-content/ uploads/2021/05/2021-05-12-The-second-wave-by-the-numbers.pdf.

102 Alexander McClelland and Alex Luscombe, "Policing the Pandemic: Counter-Mapping Policing Responses to COVID-19 across Canada," The Annual Review of Interdisciplinary Justice Research 10 (2021): 198.

103 Robyn Maynard and Andrea J. Ritchie, "Black Communities Need Support, Not a Coronavirus Police State," VICE, April 9, 2020, https://www.vice.com/en/article/ z3bdmx/black-people-coronavirus-police-state.

104   Ibid.

105   Malenfant et al., *We Can't Police Our Way Out of the Pandemic.*

106   Gary Kinsman quoted in ibid.

107   Jeffrey Ostler, "Disease Has Never Been Just Disease for Native Americans," *The Atlantic*, April 29, 2020, https://www.theatlantic.com/ideas/archive/2020/04/disease-has-never-been-just-disease-native-americans/610852/.

108   Trevor Hoppe, *Punishing Disease: HIV and the Criminalization of Sickness* (Oakland: University of California Press, 2017).

109   Maureen K. Lux, *Separate Beds: A History of Indian Hospitals in Canada, 1920s–1980s* (Toronto: University of Toronto Press, 2016).

110   Veronique Greenwood, "The Frightening Legacy of Typhoid Mary," *Smithsonian Magazine*, March 2015, https://www.smithsonianmag.com/history/the-frightening-legacy-of-typhoid-mary-180954324/.

111   Alexander McClelland, *The Criminalization of HIV Non-disclosure in Canada: Experiences of People Living with HIV in Canada*, November 21, 2019, https://www.alexandermcclelland.ca/blog-1/2019/11/21/the-criminalization-of-hiv-in-canada-experiences-of-people-living-with-hiv.

112   Ejeris Dixon and Leah Lakshmi Piepzna-Samarasinha, eds., *Beyond Survival: Strategies and Stories from the Transformative Justice Movement* (Chico, CA: AK Press, 2020).

113   This quote has been attributed to several different thinkers in the health care quality field, including Dr Paul Batalden, Dr Don Berwick, and Dr W. Edwards Deming. For more on the quote's history and origins, see Susan Carr, "A Quotation with a Life of Its Own," *Patient Safety and Quality Healthcare*, July/August 2008, https://www.psqh.com/julaug08/editor.html; Earl Conway and Paul Batalden, "Like Magic? ('Every System Is Perfectly Designed …')," Institute for Healthcare Improvement, August 21, 2015, http://www.ihi.org/communities/blogs/origin-of-every-system-is-perfectly-designed-quote.

114   T Fleischmann, *Time Is the Thing a Body Moves Through* (Minneapolis: Coffee House Press, 2019), 128.

THOUGHTS ON AN ANARCHIST RESPONSE TO HEPATITIS C AND HIV

115   Beatrice Were, "The Destructive Strings of US Aid," *New York Times*, December 15, 2005.

116   This article and larger project were initiated with the support from the Institute for Anarchist Studies though the annual Radical Writers Grant.

117 Noam Chomsky quoted in David P. Ball, "The Worst Enemy of a Government Is Its Own Population," *Indymedia Beirut*, May 13, 2006, http://beirut.indymedia .org/en/2006/05/4090.shtml.

118 UNAIDS, "Global HIV & AIDS Statistics—Fact Sheet: Preliminary UNAIDS 2021 Epidemiological Estimates," accessed June 15, 2021, https://www.unAIDS. org/en/resources/fact-sheet.

119 For further readings and analysis on HIV, housing exclusion, and regulation, see the HIV Housing Summit at http://www.hivhousingsummit.org. Also see Adrian Guta and Marilou Gagnon, "Spaces of Exclusion and Regulation: Housing Programs as Biopolitical Tools for the Management of People Living with HIV," excerpt from presentation at the 10th International Conference on New Directions in the Humanities, Montreal, Canada, June 14–16, 2012, http://h12.cgpublisher.com/proposals/198/index_html.

120 Caroline Chen, "Gilead Profit Tops Estimates as Hepatitis C Drug Sales Surge," *Bloomberg Business*, July 28, 2015, https://www.bloomberg.com/news/ articles/2015-07-28/gilead-profit-tops-estimates-as-hepatitis-c-drug-sales -surge.

121 Richard Knox, "$1,000 Pill for Hepatitis C Spurs Debate Over Drug Prices," *Health News from National Public Radio*, December 30, 2013, https://www.npr.org/ sections/health-shots/2013/12/30/256885858/-1-000-pill-for-hepatitis-c -spurs-debate-over-drug-prices.

122 Paul Barrett and Robert Langreth, "Pharma Execs Don't Know Why Anyone Is Upset by a $94,500 Miracle Cure," *Bloomberg Businessweek*, June 3, 2015, https://www.bloomberg.com/news/articles/2015-06-03/specialty-drug-costs -gilead-s-hepatitis-c-cures-spur-backlash.

123 Jason Grebely, Jesse D. Raffa, Calvin Lai, Thomas Kerr, Benedikt Fischer, Mel Kraj-den, Gregory J. Dore, and Mark W. Tyndall, "Low Uptake of Treatment for Hepatitis C Virus Infection in a Large Community-Based Study of Inner City Residents," *Journal of Viral Hepatitis* 16, no. 5 (2009): 352–58.

124 Canadian HIV/AIDS Legal Network, *The Criminalization of HIV Non-disclosure in Canada: Current Status and the Need for Change*, accessed May 24, 2021, http:// www.hivlegalnetwork.ca/site/the-criminalization-of-hiv-non-disclosure -in-canada-report/?lang=en.

125 Gary Kinsman, "Vectors of Hope and Possibility: Commentary on Reckless Vectors," *Sexuality Research & Social Policy* 2, no. 2 (2005): 99–105.

126 James C. Scott, *Two Cheers for Anarchism: Six Easy Pieces on Autonomy, Dignity, and Meaningful Work and Play* (Princeton: Princeton University Press, 2014).

127 Peter Piot, "AIDS: From Crisis Management to Sustained Strategic Response," *Lancet* 368, no. 9534 (2006): 526–30.

128   Zackie Achmat quoted in ibid.

129   Kristin Peterson, "Ethical Misrecognition: The Early PrEP Tenofovir Trial Fail-
       ures," presentation, Knowing Practices: The 2nd International Conference
       for the Social Sciences and Humanities in HIV, Paris, France, July 7–10, 2013.

130   Michael Atkin and Joel Keep, "Hep C Sufferer Imports Life Saving Drugs from
       India: Takes on Global Pharmaceutical Company," ABC News Australia,
       August 20, 2015, http://www.abc.net.au/news/2015-08-20/hepatitis-c-sufferer
       -imports-life-saving-drugs-from-india/6712990.

REGROWTH IN RUINS

131   Critical Resistance, "What Is the PIC? What Is Abolition?," accessed May 29, 2021,
       http://criticalresistance.org/about/not-so-common-language/.

132   Mariame Kaba, "So You're Thinking about Becoming an Abolitionist," in We Do
       This 'til We Free Us: Abolitionist Organizing and Transformative Justice (Chicago:
       Haymarket Books, 2021), 3.

133   Sadie Ryanne Baker quoted in Maya Schenwar and Victoria Law, Prison by Any
       Other Name: The Harmful Consequences of Popular Reforms (New York: The New
       Press, 2021), 88. Reprinted with permission.

134   Harsha Walia and Andrew Dilts, "Dismantle and Transform: On Abolition,
       Decolonization, and Insurgent Politics," Abolition: A Journal of Insurgent Pol-
       itics, May 22, 2016, https://abolitionjournal.org/dismantle-and-transform/.

135   Morgan Bassichis, Alexander Lee, and Dean Spade, "Building an Abolitionist
       Trans and Queer Movement with Everything We've Got," in Captive Genders:
       Trans Embodiment and the Prison Industrial Complex, expanded 2nd ed., eds.
       Eric A. Stanley and Nat Smith (Oakland: AK Press, 2015), 36.

136   Cameron Rasmussen and Kirk "Jae" James, "Trading Cops for Social Workers
       Isn't the Solution to Police Violence," Truthout, July 17, 2020, https://truth
       out.org/articles/trading-cops-for-social-workers-isnt-the-solution-to-police
       -violence/.

137   Stefanie Lyn Kaufman-Mthimkhulu, "We Don't Need Cops to Become Social
       Workers: We Need Peer Support + Community Response Networks," Note-
       worthy, June 6, 2020, https://blog.usejournal.com/we-dont-need-cops-to
       -become-social-workers-we-need-peer-support-b8e6c4ffe87a.

138   Jonathan Shieber, "Folx Health Raises $25 Million for Virtual Clinical Offerings
       and Care for the LGBTQIA+ Community," TechCrunch, February 2, 2021, https://
       techcrunch.com/2021/02/02/folx-health-raises-25-million-for-virtual
       -clinical-offerings-and-care-for-the-lgbtqia-community/.

139 M.V. Lee Badgett, Soon Kyu Choi, and Bianca D.M. Wilson, LGBT *Poverty in the United States: A Study of Differences between Sexual Orientation and Gender Identity Groups* (Los Angeles: The Williams Institute, 2019).

140 Niko Stratis, "Bravado and Branding: Instagrammable Startups Can't Save Trans Healthcare," *Bitch*, February 23, 2021, https://www.bitchmedia.org/article/folx-trans-healthcare-startups.

141 Katie Batza, *Before* AIDS: *Gay Health Politics in the 1970s* (Philadelphia: University of Pennsylvania Press, 2018), 5.

142 When thinking about this era, it's important to remember that 1973 was also the year homosexuality was delisted as a mental illness in the APA's *Diagnostic and Statistical Manual of Mental Disorders*.

143 Batza, *Before* AIDS, 59.

144 Alondra Nelson, *Body and Soul: The Black Panther Party and the Fight against Medical Discrimination* (Minneapolis: University of Minnesota Press, 2013).

145 Ibid.

146 Darrel Enck-Wanzer, *The Young Lords: A Reader* (New York: New York University Press, 2010).

147 Jules Gill-Peterson, "Against Transsexuality: Spirituality as Trans Feminine Practice in 1950s California," talk at the Transgender Archives, University of Victoria, January 22, 2019, https://www.youtube.com/watch?v=U8HkONpu2Jc.

148 Jules Gill-Peterson, "Greer Lankton's Living Room; or, the Occulting of Trans History," talk given at Tuning Speculation VI in Bloomington, Indiana, November 24, 2018, https://www.youtube.com/watch?v=KsbRgteMapE.

149 The ArQuives, "Rupert Raj and Trans Activism, 1971–1988," accessed May 2, 2021, https://digitalexhibitions.arquives.ca/exhibits/show/rupert-raj-and-trans-activism-/rupert-raj-and-trans-activism-.

150 Digital Transgender Archive, "Collections: *Gender Review: The* FACT*ual Newsletter*," accessed May 2, 2021, https://www.digitaltransgenderarchive.net/col/6108vb57w.

151 Cooper Lee Bombardier, *Pass with Care: Memoirs* (New York: Dottir Press, 2020), 140.

152 micha cárdenas, "Pregnancy: Reproductive Futures in Trans of Color Feminism," *Transgender Studies Quarterly* 3, nos. 1–2 (2016), 50. Reprinted with permission.

153 Doug Bierend, "Meet the GynePunks Pushing the Boundaries of DIY Gynecology," VICE, August 21, 2015, https://www.vice.com/en/article/qkvyjw/meet-the-gynepunks-pushing-the-boundaries-of-diy-gynecology.

154   Ewen Chardronnet, "GynePunk, the Cyborg Witches of DIY Gynecology," *Makery*, June 30, 2015, https://www.makery.info/en/2015/06/30/gynepunk-les
-sorcieres-cyborg-de-la-gynecologie-diy/.

155   Trans Care BC, "Who We Are," accessed March 21, 2021, http://www.phsa.ca/trans
carebc/about/who-we-are.

156   Trans Care BC, "Trans Care BC Program Update, April 2019–April 2020," accessed
March 28, 2021, http://www.phsa.ca/our-services-site/Documents/TCBC_
ProgramUpdate_2020_Final.pdf.

157   Casa de Salud, "History," accessed May 30, 2021, https://www.casadesaludnm.
org/history.

158   Ibid.

159   Casa de Salud, "Health Apprentice Program," accessed May 30, 2021, https://
www.casadesaludnm.org/volunteer.

160   Mallory Hackett, "The Role of Health Systems in Empowering Communities,"
Healthcare Finance News, February 11, 2021, https://www.healthcarefinance
news.com/news/role-health-systems-empowering-communities.

161   Anjali Taneja, interview with Autumn Brown (host), "Apocalypse Survival Skill
#8: Casa de Salud," *How to Survive the End of the World* (podcast), May 29, 2020,
https://www.endoftheworldshow.org/blog/2020/5/29/apocalypse-survival
-skill-8-casa-de-salud.

162   Casa de Salud, "History."

163   Taneja, "Apocalypse Survival Skill #8."

164   Caring for People Who Are Detained collective, *Caring for People Who Are
Detained* zine, accessed March 28, 2021, https://caringforpeople.squarespace.
com/zine.

165   Oakland Power Projects, Anti-Policing Health Toolkit, accessed March 28, 2021,
https://static1.squarespace.com/static/59ead8f9692ebee25b72f17f/t/5b6aa
b5e1ae6cfd4011275e2/1533717358865/OPP_booklet_Jun2018_v2-3.pdf.

166   MH First Oakland, "MH First Oakland: Community First Response," accessed
May 29, 2021, https://www.antipoliceterrorproject.org/mh-first-oakland.

167   Alastair Boone, "M.H. First Oakland: An Alternative to Calling the Police," *Street
Spirit*, September 1, 2020, https://thestreetspirit.org/2020/09/01/m-h-first
-oakland-an-alternative-to-calling-the-police/.

168   Devin Katayama, Ericka Cruz Guevarra, and Alan Montecillo, "What One Alternative to Policing Looks Like," KQED, June 17, 2020, https://www.kqed.org/
news/11824698/what-one-alternative-to-policing-looks-like.

169   Boone, "M.H. First Oakland."

170   Shira Hassan, interview with Cara Page and Caitlin Breedlove (hosts), "Abolition in COVID-Times: Weaving Strategies for Healing Justice and Transformative Justice," *Fortification* (podcast), August 25, 2020, https://auburnseminary.org/fortification/.

171   Zoë Dodd and Alexander McClelland, "Taking Risks Is a Path to Survival," *Developing an Anarchist Response on Hep C and HIV* (blog), July 16, 2017, https://hivhepcanarchist.tumblr.com/post/163060083647/taking-risks-is-a-path-to-survival-by-zoë-dodd. Quotations from this essay reprinted with permission.

172   Native Youth Sexual Health Network, "Frequently Asked Questions," accessed July 18, 2021, https://www.nativeyouthsexualhealth.com/nyshn-faq.

173   Billie-Jo Hardy, Alexa Lesperance, Iehente Foote, Native Youth Sexual Health Network (NYSHN), Michelle Firestone, and Janet Smylie, "Meeting Indigenous Youth Where They Are At: Knowing and Doing with 2SLGBTTQQIA and Gender Non-conforming Indigenous Youth: A Qualitative Case Study," *BMC Public Health* 20, no. 1871 (2020): doi:10.1186/s12889-020-09863-3.

174   Native Youth Sexual Health Network, *You Are Made of Medicine*, accessed July 18, 2021, https://www.nativeyouthsexualhealth.com/peersupportmanual.

175   Native Youth Sexual Health Network, "Indigenizing Harm Reduction," accessed July 18, 2021, https://www.nativeyouthsexualhealth.com/indigenizing-harm-reduction; Native Youth Sexual Health Network, "Indigenizing Harm Reduction Model," accessed July 18, 2021, https://static1.squarespace.com/static/5f3550c11c1f590e92ad30eb/t/5f45a1bfabecc042e2cadfa0/1598398915418/harmreductionmodel.pdf.

176   Native Youth Sexual Health Network, "Sexy Health Carnival," accessed July 18, 2021, https://www.nativeyouthsexualhealth.com/sexy-health-carnival.

177   Native Youth Sexual Health Network, *Sexy Health Carnival Toolkit by and for Indigenous Youth!!*, accessed July 18, 2021, https://static1.squarespace.com/static/5f3550c11c1f590e92ad30eb/t/5f45924d89367a7ca1e8a708/1598394969116/shctoolkit.pdf.

178   Native Youth Sexual Health Network, "Environmental Violence & Reproductive Justice," accessed July 18, 2021, https://www.nativeyouthsexualhealth.com/environmental-violence-reproductive-justice.

179   *Violence on the Lands, Violence on Our Bodies*, "About the Initiative," accessed May 30, 2021, http://landbodydefense.org/about/about-the-initiative.

180   ekw'í7tl Indigenous doula collective, "Our Origin Story," accessed May 29, 2021, https://ekwi7tldoulacollective.org/our-story/.

181   Danette Jubinville quoted in Zoë Ducklow and Leonardo Coelho, "Indigenous Doula Collective to Support Mother-Centred Birth Care in B.C.," *CBC News*, April 24, 2016, https://www.cbc.ca/news/aboriginal/indigenous-doula-collective-supports-mother-centred-birth-1.3546977.

182 Anna McKenzie, "Indigenous Birth Knowledge Fills Massive Gaps in Healthcare, but Needs Support," *IndigiNews*, December 4, 2020, https://indiginews.com/vancouver-island/indigenous-led-doula-training-fills-massive-gaps-in-healthcare.

183 Roberta Williams quoted in Odette Auger, "Army of Kwakwaka'wakw Doulas Bringing Birth Back Home," *IndigiNews*, November 20, 2020, https://indiginews.com/vancouver-island/army-of-kwakwakawakw-doulas-bringing-birth-back-home.

184 Matthew Green, "How PG&E's Power Shutoffs Sparked an East Bay Disability Rights Campaign," KQED, November 6, 2019, https://www.kqed.org/news/11784435/how-pges-power-shutoffs-sparked-an-east-bay-disability-rights-campaign.

185 #NoBodyIsDisposable campaign, accessed May 2, 2021, https://nobodyisdisposable.org/.

186 Robyn Maynard, "Against the Carceral State: Making (Black) Freedom in a Time of Crisis and Revolt," University of Ottawa Institute of Feminist and Gender Studies, December 3, 2020, https://www.youtube.com/watch?v=NOpRYK97IxY.

187 Dodd and McClelland, "Taking Risks Is a Path to Survival."

DREAMING BIGGER

188 Nicole C. Barbarich, "Lifetime Prevalence of Eating Disorders among Professionals in the Field," *Eating Disorders* 10, no. 4 (2002): 305–12.

189 Rebecca Earle, *The Body of the Conquistador: Food, Race and the Colonial Experience in Spanish America, 1492–1700* (New York: Cambridge University Press, 2012).

190 James W. Anderson, Elizabeth C. Konz, Robert C. Frederich, and Constance L. Wood, "Long-Term Weight-Loss Maintenance: A Meta-analysis of US Studies," *The American Journal of Clinical Nutrition* 74, no. 5 (2001): 579–84; Albert Stunkard and Mavis McLaren-Hume, "The Results of Treatment for Obesity: A Review of the Literature and Report of a Series," AMA *Archives of Internal Medicine* 103, no. 1 (1959): 79–85.

191 Your Fat Friend, "The Bizarre and Racist History of the BMI," *Elemental*, October 15, 2019, https://elemental.medium.com/the-bizarre-and-racist-history-of-the-bmi-7d8dc2aa33bb.

192 Lisa M. Brownstone, Jaclyn DeRieux, Devin A. Kelly, Lanie J. Sumlin, and Jennifer L. Gaudiani, "Body Mass Index Requirements for Gender-Affirming Surgeries Are Not Empirically Based," *Transgender Health*, published ahead of print, August 13, 2020, doi:10.1089/trgh.2020.0068.

193   Lacie L. Parker and Jennifer A. Harriger, "Eating Disorders and Disordered Eating Behaviors in the LGBT Population: A Review of the Literature," *Journal of Eating Disorders* 8, no. 1 (2020): 1–20.

194   Sara B. Kimmel and James R. Mahalik, "Body Image Concerns of Gay Men: The Roles of Minority Stress and Conformity to Masculine Norms," *Journal of Consulting and Clinical Psychology* 73, no. 6 (2005): 1185–90.

195   Elizabeth W. Diemer, Julia D. Grant, Melissa A. Munn-Chernoff, David A. Patterson and Alexis E. Duncan, "Gender Identity, Sexual Orientation, and Eating-Related Pathology in a National Sample of College Students," *Journal of Adolescent Health* 57, no. 2 (2015): 144–49.

DO YOU FEEL EMPOWERED BY YOUR JOB?

196   Ann Russo, *Feminist Accountability: Disrupting Violence and Transforming Power* (New York: NYU Press, 2018).

197   Sophie K Rosa, "Sex Workers Make Great Therapists—but They're Locked Out of the Job," *VICE*, November 9, 2019, https://www.vice.com/en/article/mbmb4y/sex-workers-therapy-profession-discrimination.

198   Phillip Cox and Aella, "Whore Phobia: The Experiences of a Dual-Training Sex Worker–Psychotherapist," *Psychotherapy and Politics International* 18, no. 2 (2020): 18:e1539, doi:10.1002/ppi.1539.

199   Butterfly (Asian and Migrant Sex Workers Support Network), *Understanding Migrant Sex Workers: Migration + Sex Work ≠ Trafficking* (Toronto: Butterfly, 2018), accessed April 2, 2021, https://576a91ec-4a76-459b-8d05-4ebbf4 2a0a7e.filesusr.com/ugd/5bd754_5826c5ca074f408988ee248d5f614219.pdf.

200   Canadian Association of Social Workers, *Decriminalization, Exit Strategies, and the Social Determinants of Health: A Three-Pronged Approach to Health, Safety and Dignity for Sex Workers. 2019 Position Statement* (Ottawa: Canadian Association of Social Workers, 2019, accessed April 2, 2021, https://www.casw-acts.ca/files/attachements/Sex_Work_Paper_Formatted_2019.pdf.

201   Stéphanie Wahab, "'For Their Own Good?': Sex Work, Social Control and Social Workers, a Historical Perspective," *Journal of Sociology and Social Welfare* 29, no. 4 (2002): 39–57.

SURVIVING TOGETHER

202   Daniel Winunwe Rivers, *Radical Relations: Lesbian Mothers, Gay Fathers, and Their Children in the United States since World War II* (Chapel Hill: University of North Carolina Press, 2013), 4.

203 Mia Birdsong, *How We Show Up: Reclaiming Family, Friendship, and Community* (New York: Hachette Books, 2020), 21.

204 Ibid., 85.

205 Victoria Law and China Martens, *Don't Leave Your Friends Behind: Concrete Ways to Support Families in Social Justice Movements and Communities* (Oakland: PM Press, 2012), 7.

206 Anna Muraco and Karen Fredriksen-Goldsen, "'That's What Friends Do': Informal Caregiving for Chronically Ill Midlife and Older Lesbian, Gay, and Bisexual Adults," *Journal of Social and Personal Relationships* 28, no. 8 (2011): 1076.

207 Elizabeth Brake, "Amatonormativity," accessed June 1, 2021, https://elizabeth brake.com/amatonormativity/

208 Angela Chen, *Ace: What Asexuality Reveals about Desire, Society, and the Meaning of Sex* (Boston: Beacon Press, 2020), 131.

209 Ibid., 132.

210 s.e. smith, "#FreeBritney Is Just the Tip of the Iceberg," *Bitch*, February 17, 2021, https://www.bitchmedia.org/article/free-britney-conservatorship-arrange ments.

211 CBC *News*, "Woman Was Illegally Detained in Hospitals for Nearly a Year, Judge Rules," February 17, 2019, https://www.cbc.ca/news/canada/british-columbia/fraser-health-detained-woman-illegally-judge-rules-1.5034179; Sasha Lakic, "Fraser Health Detained a Patient Illegally for a Year, Judge Rules," *Victoria News*, February 26, 2019, https://www.vicnews.com/news/fraser -health-detained-a-patient-illegally-for-a-year-judge-rules/.

212 As quoted in Rivers, *Radical Relations*, 118.

213 Ibid., 123.

214 Gillian Frank, "Radical Relations: An Interview with Daniel W. Rivers," *Notches* (blog), January 27, 2015, https://notchesblog.com/2015/01/27/radical-relations -an-interview-with-daniel-w-rivers/.

215 Rachel Epstein, "LGBTQ Parenting in Canada: Looking Back, Looking Forward," *LES Online* 4, no. 1 (2012), accessed April 8, 2021, https://lesonlinesite.files .wordpress.com/2017/03/lgbtq-parenting-in-canada.pdf.

216 Rivers, *Radical Relations*, 177.

217 Epstein, "LGBTQ Parenting in Canada."

218 Yasmin Nair, "Against Equality, against Marriage: An Introduction," in *Against Equality: Queer Revolution, Not Mere Inclusion*, ed. Ryan Conrad (Chico: AK Press, 2014), 21.

219 Ibid., 22.

220 Michael Waters, "Life in a Four-Mom Family," *Slate*, November 25, 2019, https://slate.com/human-interest/2019/11/queer-alternative-families-children-reflections.html.

221 Ibid.

222 Cathy J. Cohen, "Punks, Bulldaggers, and Welfare Queens: The Radical Potential of Queer Politics?," *GLQ* 3, no. 4 (1997): 453.

223 Ibid., 462.

224 Loretta J. Ross and Rickie Solinger, *Reproductive Justice: An Introduction* (Oakland: University of California Press, 2017), 9.

225 Loretta J. Ross, "Conceptualizing Reproductive Justice Theory: A Manifesto for Activism," in *Radical Reproductive Justice: Foundations, Theory, Practice, Critique*, eds. Loretta J. Ross, Lynn Roberts, Erika Derkas, Whitney Peoples, and Pamela D. Bridgewater (New York: The Feminist Press, 2017), 192.

226 Loretta Ross, "Loretta Ross of SisterSong on 'Reproductive Justice 101' Part 1," October 21, 2008, https://www.youtube.com/watch?v=JRcT_NMa6aI.

227 Kim TallBear, "On Decolonizing Sexuality through Critical Polyamory," *Strippers and Sages* (podcast interview), October 20, 2020, https://www.strippersandsages.com/kim-tallbear.

228 Scott Lauria Morgensen, "Settler Homonationalism: Theorizing Settler Colonialism within Queer Modernities," *GLQ: A Journal of Lesbian and Gay Studies* 16, no. 102 (2010): 105–31.

229 Crystal M. Hayes, Carolyn Sufrin, and Jamila B. Perritt, "Reproductive Justice Disrupted: Mass Incarceration as a Driver of Reproductive Oppression," *American Journal of Public Health* 110, no. S1 (2020): S21–S24.

230 Zsea Bowmani and Candace Bond-Theriault, *Queering Reproductive Justice: A Toolkit* (Washington: National LGBTQ Task Force, 2017), 25.

231 Ruth Dawson and Tracy Leong, "Not Up for Debate: LGBTQ People Need and Deserve Tailored Sexual and Reproductive Health Care," Guttmacher Institute, November 16, 2020, https://www.guttmacher.org/article/2020/11/not-debate-lgbtq-people-need-and-deserve-tailored-sexual-and-reproductive-health#; Abirami Kirubarajan, Priyanka Patel, Shannon Leung, Bomi Park, and Sony Sierra, "Cultural Competence in Fertility Care for Lesbian, Gay, Bisexual, Transgender, and Queer People: A Systematic Review of Patient and Provider Perspectives," *Fertility and Sterility* 115, no. 5 (2021): 1294–1301; Khadija Mitu, "Transgender Reproductive Choice and Fertility Preservation," *AMA Journal of Ethics* 18, no. 11 (2016): 1119–25.

232 Bowmani and Bond-Theriault, *Queering Reproductive Justice*, 4.

233   Alanna Vagianos, "Transgender Children across the U.S. Are Fighting for Their Lives (Again)," *Huffington Post*, April 16, 2021, https://www.huffpost .com/entry/transgender-children-fighting-for-their-lives-state-legislation _n_607881e3e4b0293a7ee00ff8?bl.

234   Lucia Leandro Gimeno, "The Reluctant Reproductive Justice Organizer and Birthworker," in *Radical Reproductive Justice*, 347–54.

235   Ruha Benjamin, "Black AfterLives Matter: Cultivating Kinfulness as Reproductive Justice," in *Making Kin Not Population*, eds. Adele E. Clarke and Donna Haraway (Chicago: University of Chicago Press, 2018), 61.

236   Kim TallBear, "Identity Is a Poor Substitute for Relating: Genetic Ancestry, Critical Polyamory, Property, and Relations," *The Critical Polyamorist* (blog), April 13, 2020, http://www.criticalpolyamorist.com/homeblog/identity-is-a -poor-substitute-for-relating-genetic-ancestry-critical-polyamory-property -and-relations.

237   Kim TaliBear, "Making Love and Relations beyond Settler Sex and Family, "in *Making Kin Not Population*, 154.

HUNGRY FOR POSSIBILITIES

235   Canadian Institute for Health Information, *The Impact of COVID-19 on Long-Term Care in Canada: Focus on the First 6 Months* (Ottawa: CIHI, 2021); *New York Times*, "Nearly One-Third of U.S. Coronavirus Deaths Are Linked to Nursing Homes," last updated April 28, 2021, https://www.nytimes.com/interactive/2020/us/ coronavirus-nursing-homes.html.

239   Liz Bradbury, "Caregiving Concerns for LGBT Older Adults," in *Bodies and Barriers: Queer Activists on Health*, eds. Adrian Shanker, Rachel L. Levine, and Kate Kendell (Oakland: PM Press, 2020), 178.

240   Ibid., 180.

241   Leah Lakshmi Piepzna-Samarasinha, *Care Work: Dreaming Disability Justice* (Vancouver: Arsenal Pulp Press, 2018).

242   Lori E. Ross and Anita Khanna, *What Are the Needs of Lesbian, Gay, Bisexual, Trans, and Queer (LGBTQ+) People That Should Be Addressed by Canada's Poverty Reduction Strategy (CPRS)?* (Toronto: Canadian Coalition Against LGBTQ+ Poverty, n.d.), accessed April 28, 2021, http://lgbtqhealth.ca/projects/docs/ prsjointsubmission.pdf.

243   Hannah Kia, "(In)Visibilities That Vary: The Production of Aging Lesbian, Gay, Bisexual, Transgender, and Queer Subjects in Chronic Care," *Theory in Action* 12, no. 3 (2019), doi:10.3798/tia.1937-0237.1919.

244 Janet Torge as quoted in CBC Radio, "Baba Yaga House, The Sequel," last modified August 10, 2013, https://www.cbc.ca/radio/sunday/baba-yaga-house-the -sequel-1.2904740?x-eu-country=false.

245 Jack Halberstam, *In a Queer Time and Place: Transgender Bodies, Subcultural Lives* (New York: NYU Press, 2005), 152.

246 Ryan Backer, personal communication to author, October 18, 2020.

247 Kai Cheng Thom, *I Hope We Choose Love: A Trans Girl's Notes from the End of the World* (Vancouver: Arsenal Pulp Press, 2019), 135.

248 Richard G. Wight, Allen J. LeBlanc, Ilan H. Meyer, and Frederick A. Harig, "Internalized Gay Ageism, Mattering, and Depressive Symptoms among Midlife and Older Gay-Identified Men," *Social Science & Medicine* 147 (2015): 200–208.

249 Ela Przybylo, *Asexual Erotics: Intimate Readings of Compulsory Sexuality* (Columbus: The Ohio State University Press, 2019), 113.

250 Sins Invalid, *Skin, Tooth, and Bone: The Basis of Movement Is Our People*, 2nd ed., 2019, 160.

251 Mia Mingus, "Interdependency (Excerpts from Several Talks)," *Leaving Evidence* (blog), January 22, 2010, https://leavingevidence.wordpress.com/ 2010/01/22/interdependency-exerpts-from-several-talks/. Reprinted with permission.

252 Erin Allday, "Last Men Standing," *San Francisco Chronicle*, March 2016, accessed April 28, 2021, https://projects.sfchronicle.com/2016/living-with-AIDS/story/.

253 Ellen Samuels, "Six Ways of Looking at Crip Time," *Disability Studies Quarterly* 37, no. 3 (2017), doi:10.18061/dsq.v37i3.5824.

254 JD Davids, Evvie Ormon, Dr Crissaris Sarnelli, and Elandria Williams, "Coronavirus: Wisdom from a Social Justice Lens," *Healing Justice Podcast*, now *Irresistible* (podcast), March 10, 2020, accessed April 29, 2021, https://docs.google. com/document/d/1sYBaoHZLQLrI8DbDbajMv2fxWOFns_sTTYUF5VTtREo/ edit?usp=sharing.

255 Katie Herzog, "Is the Life Expectancy of Trans Women in the U.S. Just 35? No.," *The Stranger*, September 23, 2019, https://www.thestranger.com/ slog/2019/09/23/41471629/is-the-life-expectancy-of-trans-women-in-the-us -just-35-no.

256 Amber Hollibaugh, interview with Caitlin Breedlove (host), *Fortification* (podcast), September 22, 2020, https://auburnseminary.org/fortification. Reprinted with permission.

257 Rose Cullis, "Don't Tell Me How to Age: On Aging, Beauty, and Expectations," *This Magazine*, September 21, 2020, https://this.org/2020/09/21/dont-tell -me-how-to-age/.

258 Jess T. Dugan and Vanessa Fabbre, *To Survive on This Shore*, accessed April 29, 2021, https://www.tosurviveonthisshore.com/.

259 Gary L. Stein, Nancy L. Beckerman, and Patricia A. Sherman, "Lesbian and Gay Elders and Long-Term Care: Identifying the Unique Psychosocial Perspectives and Challenges," *Journal of Gerontological Social Work* 53, no. 5 (2010): 421–35.

260 Kristen E. Porter, Mark Brennan-Ing, Sand C. Chang, Lore M. Dickey, Anneliese A. Singh, Kyle L. Bower, and Tarynn M. Witten, "Providing Competent and Affirming Services for Transgender and Gender Nonconforming Older Adults," *Clinical Gerontologist* 39, no. 5 (2016): 366–88.

261 Karen I. Fredriksen-Goldsen, Chengshi Shiu, Amanda E.B. Bryan, Jayn Goldsen, and Hyun-Jun Kim, "Health Equity and Aging of Bisexual Older Adults: Pathways of Risk and Resilience," *The Journals of Gerontology. Series B, Psychological Sciences and Social Sciences* 72, no. 3 (2017): 468–78.

262 Katie Tastrom, "Disability Justice and Abolition," *National Lawyers Guild*, June 27, 2020, https://www.nlg.org/disability-justice-and-abolition/.

263 United States Department of Justice Civil Rights Division, "*Olmstead*: Community Integration for Everyone," accessed April 29, 2021, https://www.ada.gov/olmstead/olmstead_about.htm.

264 Jeremy Raff, "Why Americans with Disabilities Fear Medicaid Cuts," *The Atlantic*, July 10, 2017, https://www.theatlantic.com/politics/archive/2017/07/why-disabled-american-fear-medicaid-cuts/533085/.

265 CBC *News*, "After 5 Nights in a Cage, Quebec Man Reaches Agreement with Government," August 17, 2020, https://www.cbc.ca/news/canada/montreal/chsld-jonathan-marchand-camp-national-assembly-1.5689088.

266 Linda Abbit, "Urban Cohousing the Babayaga Way," *Senior Planet*, March 6, 2016, https://seniorplanet.org/senior-housing-alternatives-urban-cohousing-the-babayaga-way/.

267 Baba Yaga Place—Toronto, website, accessed April 29, 2021, https://www.babayagaplace.ca/.

268 Rachel Covello, "All-Women's Resort in Fort Myers Is Home to 500+ Lesbians, Homes Now Available," *OutCoast*, accessed April 29, 2021, https://www.outcoast.com/carefree/.

269 KALW, "Caring for Lesbian Icon Phyllis Lyon, with Love and Deceit," June 24, 2020, https://www.kalw.org/show/crosscurrents/2020-06-24/caring-for-lesbian-icon-phyllis-lyon-with-love-and-deceit.

270 Aurora Levins Morales, homepage, accessed March 16, 2020, http://www.auroralevinsmorales.com/.

271 Aurora Levins Morales, "The Vehicle for Change," accessed March 16, 2020, http://www.auroralevinsmorales.com/vehicle-for-change.html.

272 Kinsey Clarke, "Kofi House Makes Space for Queer Women and Girls," them, March 12, 2020, https://www.them.us/story/kofi-house-queer-space.

PUT ME IN THE LIVING ROOM AND COVER ME WITH FLOWERS

273 Centre for Suicide Prevention, "Sexual Minorities and Suicide Prevention," accessed March 19, 2020, https://www.suicideinfo.ca/resource/sexual -minorities-suicide-prevention/.

274 Ibid.

275 Greg Moreau, "Police-Reported Hate Crime in Canada, 2019," Statistics Canada, March 29, 2021, https://www150.statcan.gc.ca/n1/pub/85-002-x/2021001/ article/00002-eng.htm.

276 Daniel R. Wilson, "Dying Queer in 2018," The Order of the Good Death, August 8, 2018, http://www.orderofthegooddeath.com/dying-queer-2018.

277 Sarah Chavez, "Trans Death Rights Are Human Rights," The Order of the Good Death, March 14, 2020, http://www.orderofthegooddeath.com/trans-death-rights-are-human-rights; Christine Colby, "Dying Trans: Preserving Identity in Death," The Order of the Good Death, January 10, 2017, http://www.orderof thegooddeath.com/dying-trans-preserving-identity-death.

278 Robert Cribb, Jordan Cornish, and Dale Mulligan, "Funeral Home Sales Practices Place High Cost on Grieving Families," Toronto Star, March 10, 2017, https:// www.thestar.com/news/canada/2017/03/10/funeral-home-sales-practices -place-high-cost-on-grieving-families.html; Bernhard Schroeder, "Baby Boomers Are Fueling an Industry That Is Ripe for Disruption. The Rise of the Death Concierge," Forbes, April 15, 2019, https://www.forbes.com/sites/ bernhardschroeder/2019/04/15/baby-boomers-are-fueling-an-industry-that-is -ripe-for-disruption-the-rise-of-the-death-concierge/?sh=432fe187870d.

279 Kami Fletcher, "Race & the Funeral Profession: What Jessica Mitford Missed," TalkDeath, December 2, 2018, https://www.talkdeath.com/race-funeral -profession-what-jessica-mitford-missed/.

280 Julia Calderone, "Burying Dead Bodies Takes a Surprising Toll on the Environ-ment," Business Insider, November 4, 2015, https://www.businessinsider .com/burying-dead-bodies-environment-funeral-conservation-2015-10.

281 Sophie Yeo, "Natural Burials Are Rising, and That's Good for the Planet," Pacific Standard, July 30, 2018, https://psmag.com/environment/bury-me-under -the-weeping-willow.

282 Leanna First-Arai, "Even in Death, Black Bodies Face Environmental Racism," *Truthout*, July 10, 2020, https://truthout.org/articles/even-in-death-black-bodies-face-environmental-racism/.

283 American Battlefield Trust, "Civil War Facts," last updated April 20, 2021, https://www.battlefields.org/learn/articles/civil-war-facts.

284 Brian Walsh, "When You Die, You'll Probably Be Embalmed. Thank Abraham Lincoln for That," *Smithsonian Magazine*, November 1, 2017, https://www.smithsonianmag.com/science-nature/how-lincolns-embrace-embalming-birthed-american-funeral-industry-180967038/; History.com Editors, "Abraham Lincoln's Funeral Train," last updated August 21, 2018, https://www.history.com/topics/american-civil-war/president-lincolns-funeral-train.

285 Kami Fletcher, "Feminist Death Work: A History," *Death & the Maiden*, January 24, 2018, https://deadmaidens.com/2018/01/24/feminist-death-work-a-history/.

286 Sarah Chavez, "The Story of Death Is the Story of Women," YES! *Magazine*, August 22, 2019, https://www.yesmagazine.org/issue/death/2019/08/22/dying-feminist-funeral-women-caitlin-doughty.

287 Kami Fletcher, "Decolonizing Death Studies," The Collective for Radical Death Studies, August 10, 2019, https://radicaldeathstudies.com/2019/08/10/decolonizing-death-studies/.

288 Ibid.

289 Ibid.

290 Tiffany Stanley, "The Disappearance of a Distinctively Black Way to Mourn," *The Atlantic*, January 26, 2016, https://www.theatlantic.com/business/archive/2016/01/black-funeral-homes-mourning/426807/.

291 Christine Turner, *Homegoings* (2013, PBS and Peralta Pictures), https://www.homegoings.com/.

292 Fletcher, "Race & the Funeral Profession."

293 T. Anne Richards, Judith Wrubel, and Susan Folkman, "Death Rites in the San Francisco Gay Community: Cultural Developments of the AIDS Epidemic," OMEGA: *Journal of Death and Dying* 40, no. 2 (2000): 335–50.

294 David Wojnarowicz, "Postcards from America: X Rays from Hell," in *Rebellious Mourning: The Collective Work of Grief*, ed. Cindy Milstein (Chico: AK Press, 2017), 313.

295 ACT UP New York, "The Ashes Action," accessed December 2, 2020, https://actupny.org/diva/synAshes.html.

296 ACT UP New York, "ACT UP Ashes Action 1992," https://www.youtube.com/watch?v=bWbzinqIlPk.

297   Visual AIDS, "He Would Still Be Living with AIDS," accessed April 5, 2021, https://
      visualAIDS.org/gallery/he-would-still-be-living-with-AIDS.

298   David Robinson as quoted in Sarah Schulman, *Let the Record Show: A Political
      History of ACT UP New York, 1987–1993* (New York: Farrar, Straus and Giroux,
      2021), 607.

299   ACT UP New York, "Political Funerals," accessed December 2, 2020, https://
      actupny.org/diva/polfunsyn.html.

300   Schulman, *Let the Record Show*, 618.

301   Ron Goldberg as quoted in ibid., 622.

302   Teghan Beaudette, "'Taking It to the Grave': 28-Year-Old with Terminal Cancer
      Plans Performance Art Living Funeral, "CBC News, October 11, 2016, https://
      www.cbc.ca/news/canada/manitoba/taking-it-to-the-grave-28-year-old
      -with-terminal-cancer-plans-performance-art-living-funeral-1.3799098; Jillian
      Groening, "What We Talk about When We Talk about Death," *The Dance Cur-
      rent*, October 23, 2016, https://www.thedancecurrent.com/review/what-we
      -talk-about-when-we-talk-about-death.

303   The Order of the Good Death, "Death Positive Movement," accessed March
      19, 2020, http://www.orderofthegooddeath.com/resources/death-positive
      -movement.

304   Lucinda Herring, *Reimagining Death: Stories and Practical Wisdom for Home Funer-
      als and Green Burials* (Berkeley: North Atlantic Books, 2019).

305   Kami Fletcher, interview with Susan Ruth (host), "Homegoin' and Death as Resis-
      tance," *Hey Human* (podcast), November 28, 2019, https://heyhumanpodcast
      .com/?p=3080.

306   Aisha Adkins, "Everyone Deserves a Death Buddy: The Value of Death Positive
      Friendships," The Order of the Good Death, April 27, 2019, http://www.order
      ofthegooddeath.com/everyone-deserves-a-death-buddy-the-value-of-death
      -positive-friendships.

307   Becky Burgum, "Have You Organised Your Death Party?," *Elle Magazine*, March
      12, 2020, https://www.elle.com/uk/life-and-culture/a34859744/death-party
      -funeral-trend/.

CONTRIBUTORS

Note: You can find a brief biography for each person interviewed for this book (Anita "Durt" O'Shea, Dawn Serra, Hannah Kia, Ronica Mukerjee, and Sean Saifa Wall) at the beginning of their interview.

Alexander McClelland is a settler from Toronto/Tkaronto, Ontario. He is an assistant professor at the Institute of Criminology and Criminal Justice, Carleton University. His work focuses on the intersections of life, law, and disease, where he has developed collaborative writing and academic, activist, and artistic projects to address issues of criminalization, sexual autonomy, surveillance, drug liberation, and the construction of knowledge on HIV. He has been living with HIV since 1997.

Zoë Dodd is a long-time harm reduction worker and advocate for drug user health and liberation living and working in Tkaronto/ Toronto. She spent fifteen years cofacilitating Hepatitis C support groups that are rooted in popular education and harm reduction. She was instrumental in developing a community-based model of Hep C care that prioritizes people who use drugs. She is a vocal critic of government responses to the overdose crisis; an expert in overdose response, she helped to establish Ontario's first overdose prevention site, Moss Park OPS, which ran illegally in a park for a year before receiving government funding. Zoë is a cofounder and co-organizer with the Toronto Overdose Prevention Society. She is currently working as a community scholar focused on the harms of involuntary drug treatment. She is an abolitionist and anticapitalist and is strongly committed to dismantling the drug war and the settler-colonial state of so-called "Canada."

Alexander and Zoë have been friends and collaborators for over twenty years. They have produced numerous publications and have organized together for many years.

Blyth Barnow is a minister, harm reductionist, writer, and community organizer. She was raised working class and has found community as a fat queer femme with a chronic illness. She is the founder of Femminary, an online ministry offering spiritual support for queers, femmes, people who use drugs, and harm reductionists. Every day she finds divinity in the profane, in the ordinary. Blyth graduated from Pacific School of Religion where she received a Master of Divinity and the Paul Wesley Yinger Preaching Award. She has previously contributed to *Beyond Survival: Strategies and Stories from the Transformative Justice Movement* edited by Ejeris Dixon and Leah Lakshmi Piepzna-Samarasinha.

Carly Boyce spends most of their time piecing quilts, leaving lipstick marks on taboos, and prying open binaries like oysters. They strive to be both soft and sharp and turn this energy toward their work as a therapist, facilitator, cultural producer, and community organizer. Carly is a fat femme, a genderqueer leatherdyke, an old millennial, a politicized healing worker, and an Ashkenazi Jewish witch, and knits these lineages together in their work, which hangs out in the overlapping part of the Venn diagram of personal healing and collective liberation. Their zine *helping your friends who sometimes wanna die maybe not die* (and more about their work) can be found at *tinylantern.net* and you can follow them on Instagram *@tiny.lantern*. Carly is based in Toronto/Tkaronto but maintains a long-distance romance with the Pacific.

jaye simpson is an Oji-Cree Saulteaux Indigiqueer from the Sapotaweyak Cree Nation. simpson is a writer, advocate, and activist sharing their knowledge and lived experiences in hope of creating utopia.

they are published in several magazines including *Poetry Is Dead*, *This Magazine*, PRISM *international*, SAD *Mag: Green*, GUTS magazine, *subTerrain*, *Grain*, and *Room*. they are in two anthologies: *Hustling Verse* (Arsenal Pulp Press, 2019) and *Love after the End* (Arsenal Pulp Press, 2020). *it was never going to be okay* (Nightwood Editions) is their first book of poetry, published in October 2020. It won the 2021 Indigenous Voices Award for poetry published in English, was nominated for a ReLit Award for poetry, and was a finalist for the Dayne Ogilvie Prize for LGBTQ2S+ Emerging Writers.

they are a displaced Indigenous person resisting, ruminating, and residing on xʷməθkʷəy̓əm (Musqueam), səlilwəta?ɬ (Tsleil-Waututh), and Sḵwx̱wú7mesh (Squamish) First Nations territories, colonially known as Vancouver.

Jillian Christmas is an artist, creative facilitator, curator, consultant, and advocate in the arts community. She is the long-time spoken word curator of the Vancouver Writers Fest, and former artistic director of Verses Festival of Words. Jillian has performed and facilitated workshops across North America. Winner of the 2021 Dayne Ogilvie Prize for LGBTQ2S+ Emerging Writers and the 2021 Golden Beret Award for Spoken Word Poetry, she is the author of *The Gospel of Breaking* (Arsenal Pulp Press, 2020), and the forthcoming children's book *The Magic Shell* (Flamingo Rampant, 2021). She lives on the unceded territories of the Squamish, Tsleil-Waututh, and Musqueam people (Vancouver, BC).

Joshua Wales is a queer physician and writer, with recent work in *Contemporary Verse 2* (*cv2*), *Plenitude*, *Grain*, *The New Quarterly*, the *Globe and Mail*, the *New England Journal of Medicine*, and on the CBC. He won the 2020 Peter Hinchcliffe Short Fiction Award, and his work has been shortlisted for PRISM *international's* Jacob Zilber Prize for Short Fiction, *cv2's* Young Buck Poetry Prize, and the Commonwealth Short Story Prize. He is an MFA student at UBC.

Kai Cheng Thom is a writer, performer, somatic coach, and sex educator based in Toronto/Tkaronto. She is the author of several award-winning books and an internationally known teacher of embodiment and conflict resolution.

Leah Lakshmi Piepzna-Samarasinha (she/they) is a notorious bitch who has done a lot of shit and written or coedited a lot of books, including *Beyond Survival: Stories and Strategies from the Transformative Justice Movement* (with Ejeris Dixon), *Tonguebreaker*, *Care Work: Dreaming Disability Justice*, and *Dirty River: A Queer Femme of Color Dreaming Her Way Home*. A queer disabled autistic nonbinary femme writer and disability/transformative justice worker, they are the 2020 recipient of the Lambda Foundation's Jeanne Córdova Prize for Lesbian/Queer Nonfiction, recognizing "a lifetime of work documenting the complexity of queer experience" and a 2020 Disability Futures Fellow.

Sand C. Chang, PhD, (they/them/their) is a Chinese American genderfluid/nonbinary/femme psychologist, trainer, and Body Trust Provider in practice for over fifteen years and residing on Chochenyo Ohlone land. Sand coauthored *A Clinician's Guide to Gender-Affirming Care* (New Harbinger, 2018) and the American Psychological Association's "Guidelines for Psychological Practice with Transgender and Gender Nonconforming People" (2015). Sand is a board member and section editor for *Trans Bodies, Trans Selves*, chapter author of the forthcoming WPATH SOC8, and cofounder of The Gender Affirming Letter Access Project (The GALAP), a movement to make mental health letters for trans health care financially accessible. Sand's work is focused on intersectional body liberation as it relates to trans health, sexuality, disordered eating, and somatic trauma recovery. Outside of work, Sand is a dancer, food top, punoff competitor, and small-dog enthusiast.

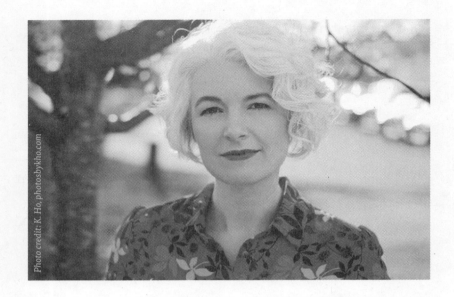

Zena Sharman (she/her) is a writer, speaker, strategist, and LGBTQ+ health advocate. Zena edited the Lambda Literary Award–winning anthology *The Remedy: Queer and Trans Voices on Health and Health Care*, and coedited the Lambda Award–nominated anthology *Persistence: All Ways Butch and Femme*, which was named a Stonewall Honor Book by the American Library Association. She regularly speaks on LGBTQ+ health to audiences of health care providers, students, and community members at universities and conferences across North America. A PhD-trained health researcher, Zena has worked in strategic leadership roles in the health research sector for over a decade. Her resumé also includes party thrower, cabaret host, go-go dancer for a queer punk band, campus radio DJ, and elementary school public speaking champion. You can learn more about Zena and her work at *zenasharman.com*.